LIVING WITH SCHIZOPHRENIA

2nd Edition

In the middle of our life's walk
I found myself alone in a dark wood
Where my path was confused

Dante, *The Divine Comedy*

LIVING WITH SCHIZOPHRENIA

2nd Edition

Dr Neel Burton

Acheron Press

Flectere si nequeo superos
Acheronta movebo

© Neel Burton 2012

Published by Acheron Press

A CIP catalogue record for this book is available from the British Library.

ISBN 978 0 9560353 7 0

Typeset by Phoenix Photosetting, Chatham, Kent, United Kingdom
Printed and bound by SRP Limited, Exeter, Devon, United Kingdom

Important notice: This is not a medical textbook and is not intended to replace advice from your doctor. Do consult your doctor if you are experiencing symptoms with which you (or others) feel that you need help.

About Neel Burton

Neel Burton is a psychiatrist and philosopher who practices and teaches in Oxford, England. He is the recipient of the Society of Authors' Richard Asher Prize, the British Medical Association's Young Authors' Award, and the Medical Journalists' Association Open Book Award. His other books include *The Meaning of Madness* and *Growing from Depression*, both also with Acheron Press.

Contents

Foreword

Unlike other medical illnesses such as heart disease, diabetes, or depression, schizophrenia is much misunderstood by the general public. Selective reporting by the media of the rare headline tragedies involving (usually untreated) schizophrenia sufferers creates the impression that they are dangerous or unpredictable. This is untrue of the vast majority, who are at greater risk of harming themselves than of harming others, and merely adds to the heavy burden of stigma that they already carry. This stigma, principally born out of ignorance, makes the day-to-day struggle against schizophrenia all the more difficult, and it is no more justified than in any other medical illness.

Living with schizophrenia can be lonely, both for sufferers and their families. By learning about the symptoms and treatments of their illness, discussing it openly, and seeking the help that is needed, they become better able to address their fears and regain personal control over their lives. This should in turn give them a better chance of leading a stable and fulfilling life and, in many cases, of making a sustained recovery.

Though information on schizophrenia is freely available in the public domain, much of it is hard to find, unreliable, inconsistent, and—because of the uncontrolled nature of the internet—unnecessarily disheartening. Much of what is easily accessible is aimed at scientists and healthcare professionals rather than at schizophrenia sufferers and their carers, for whose benefit this book has been specially prepared. By leading them to a better understanding of the illness and its treatments, from medication to psychological and other therapies, and by guiding them through their day-to-day battles, it should serve as a giant first step on their journey to recovery.

Marjorie Wallace CBE
Chief Executive, SANE

Preface

The aim of this book is to provide you and your relatives and friends with a source of information about schizophrenia that is accessible, clear, and reliable. The journey through schizophrenia is often as lonely as it is difficult, but understanding and support can do much to make it shorter, safer, and more bearable. By teaching you about schizophrenia, this book aims to allay any feelings of fear and isolation that you may have and to provide you with a realistic sense of hope and optimism. Simple and practical advice about day-to-day management enables you to take greater control over the illness, to make the most of the services that are available to you, and—ultimately—to improve your chances of once again leading a healthy, productive, and fulfilling life.

In the five years since the original edition of *Living with Schizophrenia* first came out, there have been a number of small changes in the landscape, in particular in therapeutic practices, the Mental Health Act, mental healthcare services, and social benefits. This second, fully revised edition has been prepared not only to reflect these changes, but also to build upon the surprising success of the book. For their help and advice I am indebted to Dr Phil Davison, with whom I co-authored the first edition, Marjorie Wallace, Fiona Marshall, Dr Jonathan Ray, Simon Watkins, Andrew Magee, Clare Boomer, Dr Chris Chopdar, and Dr Tom Stockmann. Any remaining errors, omissions, or deficiencies are resolutely mine.

Neel Burton

1

What's in a name? The story of schizophrenia

What does 'schizophrenia' mean?

The term 'schizophrenia' was coined in 1910 by the Swiss psychiatrist Paul Eugen Bleuler (Figure 1), and is derived from the Greek words 'schizo' (split) and 'phren' (mind). Bleuler had intended the term to refer to the dissociation or 'loosening' of thoughts and feelings that he had found to be a prominent feature of the illness.

What does 'schizophrenia' not mean?

Many people mistakenly think of schizophrenia as a 'split personality'. Robert Louis Stevenson's fictional novel *The Strange Case of Dr Jekyll and Mr Hyde* did much to popularize the concept of a 'split personality', which is sometimes also referred to as 'multiple personality disorder'. Multiple personality disorder is a vanishingly rare condition that is totally unrelated to schizophrenia. Although schizophrenia sufferers may hear voices that they attribute to various people or have strange beliefs that seem out of keeping with their usual selves, this is not the same as having a 'split personality'. Unlike Dr Jekyll, schizophrenia sufferers do not suddenly change into a different, unrecognizable person.

The term 'schizophrenia' has led to much confusion about the nature of the illness, but Bleuler had intended it to replace the older, even more misleading term of 'dementia praecox' ('dementia of early life'). This older term had been championed by the eminent German psychiatrist Emil Kraepelin, who mistakenly believed that the illness only occurred in young people and that it inevitably led to mental deterioration. Bleuler disagreed on both counts and, in an attempt to clarify matters, changed the name of the illness to 'schizophrenia'. Bleuler believed that, contrary to mental deterioration, schizophrenia led to a heightened consciousness of memories and experiences.

It is as common as it is unfortunate to hear the adjective 'schizophrenic' being bandied about to mean 'changeable' or 'unpredictable'. This usage should be discouraged because it perpetuates people's misunderstanding of the illness and

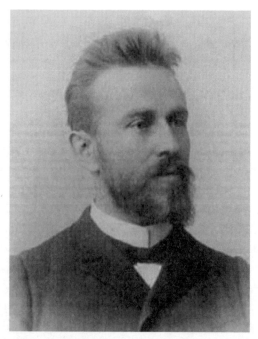

Figure 1:   Paul Eugen Bleuler (1857–1940).

contributes to the stigmatization of schizophrenia sufferers. Even used correctly, the term 'schizophrenic' does little more than label a person according to an illness, implicitly diminishing him or her to little more than that illness. For this reason, I have dropped the term 'schizophrenic' from this book in favour of 'schizophrenia sufferer'. A person is not a 'schizophrenic' any more than he or she is a 'diabetic' or suffering with toothache.

Who 'discovered' schizophrenia?

Although Kraepelin had some mistaken beliefs about the nature of schizophrenia, he was the first person to distinguish the illness from other forms of psychosis, and in particular from the 'affective psychoses' that occur in mood disorders such as depression and manic-depressive illness (bipolar affective disorder). His classification of mental disorders, the *Compendium der Psychiatrie*, is the forerunner of the two most influential classifications of mental disorders, the International Classification of Diseases 10th Revision (ICD-10) and the Diagnostic and Statistical Manual of Mental Disorders 4th revision (DSM-IV). Today these classifications are principally based on scientific research and expert opinion and, particularly in the case of ICD-10, on international consultation and consensus. As well as listing mental disorders, they provide operational definitions and diagnostic criteria that doctors use to reach a diagnosis of schizophrenia (see Chapter 4).

Kraepelin first isolated schizophrenia from other forms of psychosis in 1887, but this is not to say that schizophrenia— or 'dementia praecox', as he called it—had not existed long before Kraepelin's day. The oldest available description of an illness closely resembling schizophrenia can be found in the Ebers papyrus, which dates back to the Egypt of 1550 BC. And archaeological discoveries of Stone Age skulls with burr holes drilled into them (presumably to release 'evil spirits') have led to speculation that schizophrenia is as old as mankind itself.

How was schizophrenia thought of in antiquity?

In antiquity, people did not think of 'madness' (a term that they used indiscriminately for all forms of psychosis) in terms of mental illness, but in terms of divine punishment or demonic possession. Evidence for this comes from the Old Testament and most notably from the First Book of Samuel, according to which King Saul became 'mad' after neglecting his religious duties and angering God. The fact that David used to play on his harp to make Saul better suggests that, even in antiquity, people believed that psychotic illnesses could be successfully treated.

> But the spirit of the Lord departed from Saul, and an evil spirit from the Lord troubled him … And it came to pass, when the evil spirit from God was upon Saul, that David took an harp, and played with his hand: so Saul was refreshed, and was well, and the evil spirit departed from him. —1 Samuel 16.14, 16.23 (KJV)

When did people first start thinking of schizophrenia as an illness?

In Greek mythology and the Homerian epics, madness is similarly thought of as a punishment from God—or the gods— and it is in actual fact not until the time of the Greek physician Hippocrates (460–377 BC) that mental illness first became an object of scientific speculation. Hippocrates thought that madness resulted from an imbalance of four bodily humours and that it could be cured by rebalancing these humours with such treatments as special diets, purgatives, and blood-lettings. To modern readers, Hippocrates' ideas may seem far-fetched, perhaps even on the dangerous side of eccentric, but in the fourth century BC they represented a significant advance on the idea of mental illness as a punishment from God. The Greek philosopher Aristotle (384–322 BC) and later the Roman physician Galen (129–216) expanded on Hippocrates' humoral theories and both men played an important role in establishing them as Europe's dominant medical model.

> *Only from the brain springs our pleasures, our feelings of happiness, laughter and jokes, our pain, our sorrows and tears … This same organ makes us mad or confused, inspires us with fear and anxiety…* —Hippocrates, *The Holy Disease*

It is perhaps worth noting that not everybody in antiquity invariably thought of 'madness' as a curse or an illness. In Plato's *Phaedrus*, the Greek philosopher Socrates (470–399 BC) says,

> *Madness, provided it comes as the gift of heaven, is the channel by which we receive the greatest blessings … the men of old who gave things their names saw no disgrace or reproach in madness; otherwise they would not have connected it with the name of the noblest of arts, the art of discerning the future, and called it the manic art … So, according to the evidence provided by our ancestors, madness is a nobler thing than sober sense … madness comes from God, whereas sober sense is merely human.*

In Ancient Rome, the physician Asclepiades and the statesman, philosopher, and writer Cicero (106–43 BC) rejected Hippocrates' humoral theories, asserting, for example, that melancholia (depression) resulted not from an excess of 'black bile' but from emotions such as rage, fear, and grief. Unfortunately, in the first century AD the influence of Asclepiades and Cicero began to decline, and the influential Roman physician Celsus reinstated the idea of madness as a punishment from the gods—an idea to be later reinforced by the rise of Christianity and the collapse of the Roman Empire. In the Middle Ages, religion became central to cure and, alongside the mediaeval asylums such as the Bethlehem in London, some monasteries transformed themselves into centres for the treatment of mental illness. This is not to say that the humoral theories of Hippocrates had been forgotten, but merely that they had been incorporated into the prevailing Christian beliefs, and the purgatives and blood-lettings continued alongside the prayers and confession.

How did beliefs change?

The burning of the so-called heretics—often people suffering from psychotic illnesses such as schizophrenia—began in the early Renaissance and reached its peak in the fourteenth and fifteenth centuries. First published in 1563, *De praestigiis daemonum* (The Deception of Demons) argued that the madness of 'heretics' resulted not from divine punishment or demonic possession, but from natural causes. The Church forbade the book and accused its author, Johann Weyer, of being a sorcerer. From the fifteenth century, scientific breakthroughs such as those of the astronomer Galileo (1564–1642) and the anatomist Vesalius (1514–1584) began challenging the authority of the Church, and the centre of attention and study gradually shifted from God to man and from the heavens to the Earth. Unfortunately, this did not immediately translate into better treatments, and Hippocrates' humoral theories persisted up to and into the eighteenth century. Empirical thinkers such as John Locke (1632–1704) in England and Denis Diderot (1713–1784) in France challenged this status quo by arguing, very much as Cicero had done, that reason and emotions are caused by nothing more or less than sensations. Also in France, the physician Philippe Pinel (1745–1826) began regarding mental illness as the result of exposure to psychological and social stressors. A landmark in the history of psychiatry, Pinel's *Medico-Philosophical Treatise on*

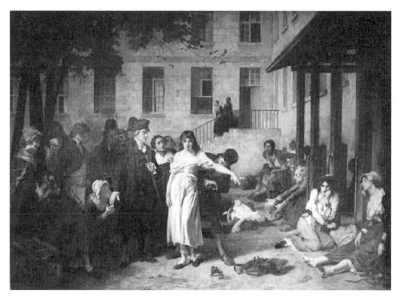

Figure 2:   In this 1876 painting by Tony Robert-Fleury, Pinel is seen freeing people with mental illness from the confinements of the old asylums. (Charcot Library, Salpêtrière Hospital Medical School, Paris.)

Mental Alienation or Mania called for a more humane approach to the treatment of mental illness. This so-called 'moral treatment' included respect for the person, a trusting and confiding doctor-patient relationship, decreased stimuli, routine activity, and the abandonment of old-fashioned Hippocratic treatments (Figure 2). At about the same time as Pinel in France, the Tukes (father and son) in England founded the York Retreat, the first institution 'for the humane care of the insane' in the British Isles.

How did beliefs evolve in the 20th century?

The founder of psychoanalysis, the Viennese psychiatrist Sigmund Freud (1856–1939), influenced much of twentieth century psychiatry. As a result of his influence, by the second half of the twentieth century the majority of psychiatrists in the USA (although not in the UK) believed that schizophrenia resulted from unconscious conflicts originating in childhood.

Since then, the advent of antipsychotic medication, advanced brain imaging, and molecular genetic studies has confirmed beyond any reasonable doubt that schizophrenia is a biological disease of the brain.

Yet it is also recognized that psychological and social stresses can play an important role in triggering episodes of illness, and that different approaches to treatment should be seen not as competing but as complementary. Thanks to this fundamental realization, the advent of antipsychotic medication, and the shift to care in the community, schizophrenia sufferers today stand a better chance than ever before of leading a healthy, productive, and fulfilling life.

What treatments were used before the advent of antipsychotic medication?

Febrile illnesses such as malaria had been observed to temper psychotic symptoms, and in the early twentieth century 'fever therapy' became a common form of treatment for schizophrenia. Psychiatrists tried to induce fevers in their patients, sometimes by means of injections of sulphur or oil. Other popular but unsatisfactory treatments included sleep therapy, gas therapy, electroconvulsive or electroshock treatment, and prefrontal leucotomy—the removal of the part of the brain that processes emotions. Sadly, many such 'treatments' were aimed more at controlling disturbed behaviour than at curing illness or alleviating suffering. In some countries, such as Germany during the Nazi era, the belief that schizophrenia resulted from a 'hereditary defect' even led to atrocious acts of forced sterilization and genocide. The first antipsychotic drug, chlorpromazine, first became available in the 1950s (see Chapter 7), and opened up an era of hope and promise for schizophrenia sufferers and their carers. Since the advent of antipsychotic drugs, the use of electroconvulsive therapy in schizophrenia has become increasingly rare. Nevertheless, it should be underlined that modern electroconvulsive therapy is a safe and humane intervention, and that it can be highly effective in the treatment of severe mood symptoms that have not responded to medication.

So, where to now?

In 1919, Kraepelin stated that 'the causes of dementia praecox are at the present time still mapped in impenetrable darkness'. Since then, greater understanding of the causes of schizophrenia has opened up multiple avenues for the prevention and treatment of the illness, and a broad range of pharmacological, psychological, and social interventions have been scientifically proven to work.

Today, schizophrenia sufferers stand a better chance than at any other time in history of leading a normal life. And thanks to the fast pace of on-going medical research, a good outcome is increasingly likely.

2

Who is affected by schizophrenia, and why?

Many schizophrenia sufferers and their families do not talk openly about the illness for fear of being misunderstood or stigmatized. This deplorable state of affairs can lead to the impression that schizophrenia is very rare.

In fact, schizophrenia is so common that most people will know of someone with the illness.

The chance of any given person developing schizophrenia in his or her lifetime is about 1 per cent or 1 in 100; and the chance of any given person suffering from schizophrenia at any one time is 0.4 per cent or 1 in 250.

Why is such a terrible illness so common?

Genes for potentially debilitating illnesses usually become less common over time: the fact that this hasn't happened for schizophrenia suggests that the responsible genes are being selected despite their potentially debilitating effects on a significant proportion of the population. The reason for this could be that the genes confer important adaptive advantages to our species, such as the abilities for language and creativity. Our abilities for language and creativity not only set us clearly apart from other animals, but also make us highly adept at the game of survival—an idea that I discuss at much greater length in my book, *The Meaning of Madness*.

Schizophrenia and creativity

Some highly creative people have suffered from schizophrenia, including Syd Barrett, the early driving force behind the rock band Pink Floyd; John Nash, the father of 'game theory' and Nobel Prize winner; and Vaslav Nijinsky, the legendary choreographer and dancer. It must be stressed that such people are at their most creative not during active phases of illness but before the onset of the illness and during later phases of remission.

Similarly, many highly creative people have had close relatives who have been affected by schizophrenia, such as the physicist Albert Einstein (his son), the philosopher Bertrand Russell (also his son), and the novelist James Joyce (his daughter). Studies have suggested that this may not be simple coincidence, and that the relatives of schizophrenia sufferers benefit from above average creative intelligence.

At what age does schizophrenia present?

Schizophrenia can present at any age, but is rare in childhood and early adolescence. Most cases are diagnosed in late adolescence or early adulthood. If symptoms indicative of schizophrenia occur for the first time in middle or old age, it is particularly important for the psychiatrist to exclude other conditions that can present like schizophrenia (see Table 5 in Chapter 4). This is not only because such conditions are more common in older people, but also because it is unusual for schizophrenia to develop so late in life.

Is schizophrenia equally common in men and women?

Schizophrenia affects men and women in more or less equal numbers. However, the illness tends to present at a younger age in men, and also tends to affect men more severely. Why this should be still remains unclear. Note that this is not a rule but a trend, and that many men with schizophrenia go on to make a complete or near-complete recovery.

Is schizophrenia equally common in all cultures and ethnic groups?

Schizophrenia exists in all cultures and ethnic groups, but—perhaps surprisingly—its outcome tends to be more favourable in developing countries than in developed countries. This is thought to be because traditional and tight-knit communities such as those typically found in developing countries are more tolerant of mental illness and better able to care for and support their mentally ill. This is important because it suggests that attitudes of family and friends can make an important difference to the outcome of the illness.

Is schizophrenia equally common in urban and rural environments?

Schizophrenia tends to be more common in inner cities and urban areas than in rural areas. The reasons for this are unclear: it could be that the stress of urban life increases the risk of developing the illness (the so-called 'breeder hypothesis'), or that people with the illness have an overall tendency to migrate out of rural areas and into urban areas (the 'drift hypothesis')—or perhaps both.

Why does schizophrenia affect some people and not others?

There is no one gene that can be said to cause schizophrenia. Rather, there are several genes that are independent of one another and that, cumulatively, make a person more or less vulnerable to developing the illness. A person who is highly vulnerable to developing schizophrenia but who is never subjected to severe stress may be less likely to develop or express the illness than a person who is only moderately vulnerable but who comes under severe stress (Figure 3). Examples of severe stress are losing a friend or relative in an accident, being badly bullied at school, or smoking cannabis (a form of physical, as opposed to emotional, stress).

The situation is analogous to that of many other important conditions such as heart disease or diabetes. Taking heart disease as an example, every person inherits a certain complement of genes that make him or her more or less vulnerable to developing the illness. Regardless of this vulnerability, if he or she maintains a healthy diet, takes regular exercise, and drinks in moderation, then he or she is likely to remain healthy.

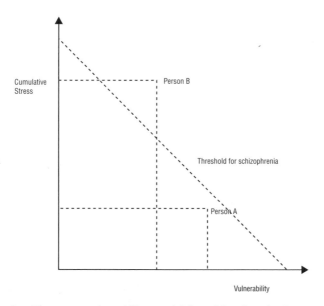

Figure 3:   The stress-vulnerability model for schizophrenia. A person develops schizophrenia when the stress that he faces becomes greater than his ability to cope with it. Person A is highly vulnerable to developing schizophrenia but is only ever subjected to moderate stress and thus never develops the illness. Person B in contrast, though less vulnerable, is subjected to such severe stress that it carries him beyond his threshold for developing the illness.

The role of genes in schizophrenia

If a person with an identical twin (that is, a twin who shares exactly the same genes) develops schizophrenia, the chance of the other identical twin also developing the illness is about 50 per cent or one in two. What this says is that genes do play an important role in the causation of schizophrenia, but that they are not the whole story. If genes were the whole story, then the chance of the identical twin also developing the illness would be 100 per cent. The fact that the figure is 'only' 50 per cent tells us that, in the causation of schizophrenia, genes are quite literally only half the story.

From Figure 4, it is apparent that a person's family history of schizophrenia is an important determinant of his or her risk of developing the illness. If a person has no family history of schizophrenia, then his or her lifetime risk of developing the illness is less than one per cent —a risk, as might be expected,

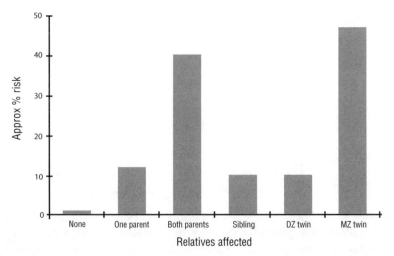

Figure 4: Lifetime risks of schizophrenia according to which relatives are affected. MZ twin, identical twin (a twin who shares exactly the same genes); DZ twin, non-identical twin (a twin who shares only half the same genes, like any other sibling).

broadly similar to that of the general population. However, if a person has a parent or sibling who has been affected by schizophrenia, then his or her lifetime risk of developing the illness rises to about, respectively, 12 per cent and 10 per cent. These figures are only average figures, because many factors other than family history are involved in determining a person's lifetime risk of developing schizophrenia. Although there is not much that a person can do about his or her family history, there is a lot that he or she can do about these other, so-called 'environmental', factors.

The role of environmental factors in schizophrenia

As dictated by the stress-vulnerability model (see Figure 3), a person develops schizophrenia if the amount of stress that he or she comes under exceeds his or her genetically determined ability to cope with it. This stress is often related to so-called life events, that is, important events such as losing a loved one, going through a divorce or separation, losing a job, or falling ill. Though life events need not be negative, they are invariably perceived as being highly stressful. Thus, events such as getting married, having a baby, or even going on holiday can count as significant life events for certain people. The corollary here is that life events are subjective: a life event for me is not necessarily a life event for you, and vice versa.

From Figure 5, it can be seen that, on the one hand, life events can precipitate schizophrenia and that, on the other, schizophrenia—or its early or prodromal phase (see chapter 3)—can precipitate life events. For example, if a person in the prodromal phase is experiencing difficulty in concentrating, confusion, and lack of energy, then he is more likely to lose

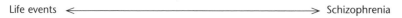

Life events ⟵————————————————————⟶ Schizophrenia

Figure 5:   The relationship between life events and schizophrenia.

his job than the average person. Moreover, the stress induced by losing his job may be great enough to tip him over into schizophrenia. So as you can see, the relationship between life events and schizophrenia is far from being a simple one.

Although life events can cause a lot of stress, it is important to highlight that most of the stress that a person experiences on a daily basis comes not from life events, but from seemingly smaller 'background' stressors such as tense relationships, painful memories (especially memories of physical or sexual abuse), isolation, discrimination, poor housing, or unpaid bills. The cumulative effect of these stressors can be far greater than that of any single life event and may alone be sufficient to tip a person into schizophrenia.

A final point about stress, implicit in the stress-vulnerability model (see Figure 3), is that different people are able to handle different amounts of stress. The amount of stress that a given person is able to handle is related to his genetic vulnerability to schizophrenia, but also to his thinking and coping styles and ability and opportunities for social interaction.

People with positive coping and thinking styles and good social skills are better able to diffuse stressful situations—for example, by doing something about them, putting them in their proper context, or simply talking about them and 'sharing the pain'. Again, the relationship between coping and thinking styles and vulnerability to schizophrenia is far from being a simple one, as people with a high vulnerability to schizophrenia are also more likely to have poorer coping and thinking styles.

The concept of 'expressed emotion'

Expressed emotion can be thought of as a specific type of stress. It refers to the amount of critical, hostile, or emotionally over-involved attitudes directed at the schizophrenia sufferer by his or her carers. Such attitudes often originate in a misunderstanding that the schizophrenia sufferer is actually in control of his or her illness and 'choosing' to be ill. Alternatively, over-involvement can result from an unjustified sense of guilt about the schizophrenia sufferer's illness, and a desire on the part of the carer to 'share out' the suffering. A number of studies have demonstrated that high expressed emotion is an important risk factor for relapse in schizophrenia, and that it can increase the risk of relapse by up to 4 times. High expressed emotion from carers may lead a schizophrenia sufferer to feel trapped, helpless, and/or guilty, and the stress of all this may lead to a relapse of the illness. As with the relationship between life events and schizophrenia, the relationship between expressed emotion and schizophrenia is far from being a simple one.

Figure 6 demonstrates that high expressed emotion can precipitate a relapse of schizophrenia, but also that it can reflect legitimate feelings of anxiety and distress induced by illness in a loved one. It cannot be stressed enough that parents should not blame themselves for their son or daughter's illness. Instead, they should remember that they are their child's most valuable source of structure and support, and his or her greatest hope for a permanent recovery.

High expressed emotion 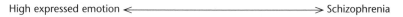 Schizophrenia

Figure 6:   The relationship between high expressed emotion and schizophrenia.

Cannabis and other drugs

Many people with schizophrenia turn to alcohol or illicit drugs such as cannabis, amphetamines, or cocaine to obtain relief from their symptoms and associated feelings of anxiety and depression. These substances might temporarily blunt or mask their symptoms, but in the long term may lead to more frequent and severe relapses of the illness. They may also delay getting help, including getting an all-important prescription for antipsychotic medication.

Research has found that **people who smoke cannabis are up to 6 times more likely to develop schizophrenia**, and that people with schizophrenia who smoke cannabis have more frequent and more severe relapses of the illness. This does not necessarily mean that cannabis causes schizophrenia, just as the association between red wine and cardiovascular fitness does not necessarily mean that red wine prevents heart disease (it could be, for example, that people who drink red wine also have healthier lifestyles). However, from what we know about how cannabis affects the brain, it seems highly likely that the drug can precipitate a first or subsequent episode of schizophrenia. For this reason, counselling about cannabis use can be an important part of a schizophrenia sufferer's care plan.

Other drugs that have been associated with schizophrenia include stimulant drugs such as amphetamines, ecstasy, and cocaine.

Other possible factors

People born between the months of January and April have a 5–10 per cent increased chance of developing schizophrenia. This increased chance is referred to as the 'season-of-birth effect', and is thought to reflect the higher risk of viral infections during the winter season. The season of birth effect provides some support to the theory that events taking place before or at the time of birth can exert an influence on a person's later vulnerability to developing schizophrenia.

Similarly, there is some limited evidence to suggest that obstetric complications (complications during pregnancy and at the time of delivery) can also increase the risk of the child later developing schizophrenia.

In conclusion

It appears that a person's risk of developing schizophrenia depends primarily on his or her genetic makeup. However, this risk may not be actualized unless the person experiences a higher level of stress than he or she can cope with. This stress may be both a cause *and* a consequence of his or her illness. For example, a person in the early prodromal phase may no longer be able to concentrate adequately and, as a result, may lose his or her job. The resulting stress may then push him or her beyond the threshold for developing the illness. As you can see, this interplay of genetic and environmental factors is far from being simple.

3

Symptoms

The symptoms of schizophrenia are manifold, and present in such a variety of combinations and severities that it is impossible to describe a 'typical case' of schizophrenia. In the short term, symptoms may wax and wane, with the schizophrenia sufferer experiencing both good days and bad days. In the long term, the emphasis may shift from one group of symptoms to another, presenting different challenges for the schizophrenia sufferer and his or her carers.

The symptoms of schizophrenia are usually divided into three groups: positive symptoms, cognitive symptoms, and negative symptoms, as listed in Table 1.

Table 1:   Symptoms of schizophrenia

Positive symptoms
Hallucinations
Delusions
Cognitive symptoms
Difficulties with attention, concentration and memory
Negative symptoms
Restricted range of emotions, or inappropriate emotions
Loss of drive and motivation
Social withdrawal
Restricted amount and/or range of thought and speech
Impaired attention

Each of these symptoms is fully explained in this chapter

Positive symptoms

Positive symptoms consist of psychotic symptoms (hallucinations and delusions), which are usually as real to the schizophrenia sufferer as they are unreal to everybody else. Positive symptoms are usually considered to be the hallmark of schizophrenia, and are often most prominent in the early stages of the illness. They can be provoked or aggravated by stressful situations, such as succumbing to a physical illness, breaking off a relationship, or leaving home to go to university.

Hallucinations

Psychiatrists define a hallucination as 'a sense perception that arises in the absence of a stimulus'. Hallucinations involve hearing,

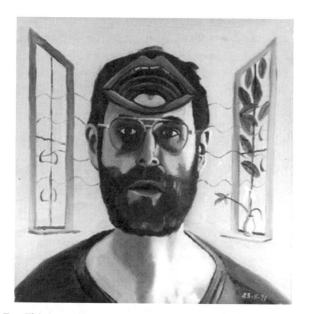

Figure 7:   This is a self-portrait of a schizophrenia sufferer who appears to be hearing his own thoughts as if they are being spoken aloud. This is a special form of auditory hallucination referred to as 'thought echo' (SANE/ Bryan Charnley).

seeing, smelling, tasting, or feeling things that are not actually there. The most common hallucinations in schizophrenia are auditory hallucinations—hallucinations of sounds and voices. Voices can either speak *to* the schizophrenia sufferer (second-person, 'you' voices) or *about* him (third-person, 'he' voices). Voices can be highly distressing, especially if they involve threats or abuse, or if they are loud and incessant. (Carers might begin to experience something of the distress of hearing voices by turning on both the radio and the television at the same time, both at full volume, and then trying to hold a normal conversation.) On the other hand, some voices—such as the voices of old acquaintances, dead ancestors, or 'guardian angels'—can be a source of comfort and reassurance rather than of distress.

Delusions

Delusions are defined as 'strongly held beliefs that are not amenable to logic or persuasion and that are out of keeping with their holder's background'. Although delusions need not necessarily be false, the process by which they are arrived at is usually bizarre and illogical. In schizophrenia, delusions are most often of being persecuted or controlled, although they can also follow a number of other themes. Common delusional themes and some examples of each are listed in Table 2.

Table 2: Delusional themes in schizophrenia

Delusional theme	Explanation
Delusions of persecution	Delusions of being persecuted – for example, being spied upon by secret services or being poisoned by aliens
Delusions of control	Delusions that one's feelings, thoughts or actions are being controlled by an external force – for example, having one's thoughts 'stolen' by aliens and replaced by different thoughts

Delusional theme	Explanation
Delusions of reference	Delusions that objects, events or other persons have a particular and unusual significance relating to the self – for example, receiving a series of coded messages from the aliens while listening to a programme on Radio 4
Delusions of grandeur	Delusions of being invested with special status, a special purpose or special abilities – for example, being the most intelligent person on earth and having the responsibility of saving it from the effects of climate change. Delusions of grandeur are more common in manic psychosis (bipolar affective disorder) than in schizophrenia
Religious delusions	Delusions of having a special relationship with God or a supernatural force – for example, being the next messiah, or being persecuted by the devil
Delusions of guilt	Delusions of having committed a crime or having sinned greatly – for example, being personally responsible for a recent tourist attack and therefore deserving severe punishment
Nihilistic delusions	Delusions that one no longer exists or is about to die or suffer a personal catastrophe. In some cases there may be a belief that other people or objects no longer exist or that the world is coming to an end. Nihilistic delusions are more common in depressive psychosis (a severe form of depression) than in schizophrenia
Somatic delusions	Delusions of being physically ill or having deformed body parts
Delusions of jealousy	Delusions that one's spouse or partner has been unfaithful
Delusions of love	Delusions of being loved by someone who is inaccessible or with whom one has little contact
Delusions of misidentification	Delusions that familiar people have been replaced by identical-looking imposters (Capgras delusion), or that they are disguising as various strangers (Fregoli delusion)

Case study

Robert Bayley, a schizophrenia sufferer who has chosen to publicly discuss his illness, writes about his experience of auditory and visual hallucinations.

As I open my eyes to greet a new day, voices commence with their attack—voices that discuss and ridicule my every move and thought, as though they can be heard from another room. They deride me, breaking down any feelings of positivity, gaining in momentum, reaching the very core of my mind. I also hear an officious, commanding voice that issues instructions, his vocalization resembling an automaton. Together they resonate and modulate, growing in their penetration, until they can be heard screaming. I also hear strange atonal sounds, and they in turn become akin to cacophony. As I rise from my slumber, the scenarios become more complex, as theatrical scenes are played out, and I hear all the individual characters reading out their lines from differing areas and locations inside the brain. Then these slowly dissipate, and I am left with the paranoid reality that is created by the automaton and the destroyers of Faith.

The next manifestation appears, as glistening beams descend from the ceiling, and the walls begin to close in. Objects inanimate are injected with life, and they gyrate and flex, as the floor ripples like the agitated flow of a river. I have spent hours transfixed by items of furniture that have conversed with me, as though possessing their own spirit, moving around without effort. Also, familiar people are translated into other forms, such as my wife into a painting or ornament. Demonic faces erupt from the group, shattering in front of my petrified eyes. Existence becomes increasingly paranoid, as feelings of fear encompass, until the desire to mutilate can rear its ugly head, just to attain that sensation of release. Vast blocks of ominous tones hover over me, only to descend, as the ceilings come crashing down.

I have spent so many hours existing within a world where actuality cannot easily be defined. I enter different dimensions, places where terror resides, a waking nightmare. As I endeavour to look outwards, my vision fragments into a thousand little pieces. I am left to put it all back together.

Is a person with positive symptoms dangerous or unpredictable?

Positive symptoms correspond to the general public's conception of 'madness', and people with prominent hallucinations or delusions may evoke fear and anxiety in others. Such feelings are often reinforced by selective reporting by the media of the rare headline tragedies involving people with (usually untreated) mental illness. The reality is that the vast majority of schizophrenia sufferers are no more likely than the average person to pose a risk to others, but far more likely than the average person to pose a risk to themselves. For example, they may neglect their safety and personal care, or they may leave themselves open to emotional, physical, or financial exploitation.

How can carers best deal with positive symptoms?

Positive symptoms can be very distressing, both to the schizophrenia sufferer and to his or her carers. Carers often find themselves challenging the schizophrenia sufferer's hallucinations and delusions, partly out of a desire to relieve his or her suffering, and partly out of understandable feelings of fear and helplessness. Unfortunately this can be counterproductive, because it can alienate the schizophrenia sufferer from his or her carers at the very time that he or she needs them most. Difficult though this may be, carers should not lose sight of the fact that positive symptoms are as real to the schizophrenia sufferer as they are unreal to everybody else.

A more helpful course of action for carers is to recognize that the schizophrenia sufferer's hallucinations and delusions are real and important to him or her, whilst making it clear that they do not personally share in them. For example,

Person: *The aliens are telling me that they are going to abduct me tonight.*
Carer: *That sounds terribly frightening.*
P: *I've never felt so frightened in all my life.*
C: *I can understand that you feel frightened, although I myself can't hear the aliens you speak of.*
P: *You mean, you can't hear them?*
C: *No, not at all. Have you tried ignoring them?*
P: *If I listen to my iPod they don't seem so loud, and I feel a bit more calm.*
C: *What about when we talk together, like now?*
P: *That's very helpful too.*

Cognitive symptoms

Cognitive symptoms involve problems with concentration and memory that can cause difficulty understanding conversation, registering and recalling information, and thinking and expressing thoughts. Cognitive symptoms are often detectable in the prodromal phase of schizophrenia before the onset of positive symptoms and, though less evident than positive symptoms, can be just as distressing and disabling. Compared with positive symptoms, cognitive symptoms are less responsive to antipsychotic medication (see Chapter 7).

Negative symptoms

Whereas positive symptoms can be thought of as an excess or distortion of normal functions, negative symptoms can be thought of as a diminution or loss of normal functions. Compared with positive symptoms, negative symptoms tend to be more subtle and less noticeable but also more persistent. Indeed, they can remain even through periods of remission, long after any positive symptoms have burnt out or faded into the background.

Negative symptoms can be difficult to pinpoint and, sadly, are often misconstrued by the general public—and sometimes also by relatives and carers—as laziness or obstreperousness. For healthcare professionals, negative symptoms can sometimes be difficult to differentiate from symptoms of depression, which are common in schizophrenia, or from certain of the side effect of antipsychotic medication.

As previously discussed, schizophrenia can present in such a variety of combinations and severities that it is impossible to describe a 'typical case' of schizophrenia. In some cases, negative symptoms can dominate the illness; in others they may be altogether absent. During periods of remission, the severity of any residual negative symptoms is an important determinant of the schizophrenia sufferer's overall quality of life and ability to function.

Negative symptoms are listed in Table 3. Compared with positive symptoms, and like cognitive symptoms, they tend to be poorly responsive to antipsychotic medication.

Table 3: Negative symptoms in schizophrenia

Negative symptom	Explanation
Restricted range of emotions or inappropriate emotions	Appearing flat and unresponsive to circumstances and events, or responding to them inappropriately
Loss of drive and motivation	Finding it difficult to do things such as cleaning, shopping, or participating in leisure activities. In more severe cases, being unable to fulfil basic needs such as bathing, grooming and feeding. Schizophrenia sufferers are sometimes accused of being 'lazy', but this is unfair as loss of drive and motivation can be symptoms of the illness

Table 3 – *continued*

Negative symptom	Explanation
Social withdrawal	Finding it difficult to make friends or hold on to old friendships, resulting in a lack of intimate relationships
Poverty of thought and speech	Experiencing a marked reduction in the amount and complexity of thinking, and finding thinking to be difficult and tiring. Poverty of thought usually manifests itself as poverty of speech, involving restricted verbal interaction and a lack of spontaneous speech. For example, replies to questions may principally consist of stock phrases (such as, 'Oh dear, that's not good') and other short sentences
Impaired attention	Not being able to focus the attention for any length of time, thereby finding it difficult to take in information and complete tasks

How do the symptoms of schizophrenia change over time?

The course of schizophrenia can vary considerably from one person to the next, but is often marked by a number of distinct phases (Figure 8). In the acute (or 'initial and short-lasting') phase, positive symptoms come to the fore, while any cognitive and negative symptoms that may already be present appear to sink into the background. The schizophrenia sufferer typically reaches a crisis point when contact with mental health services is made. Antipsychotic medication is started and the acute phase resolves, even though residual positive symptoms may still remain in the background for some time. As the acute phase resolves, the cognitive and negative symptoms may return to the fore and dominate the picture. This chronic (or 'long-lasting') phase, if it occurs, may last for a period of several months or, in some cases, several years, and may be punctuated by relapses into a condition resembling the acute phase. Common causes

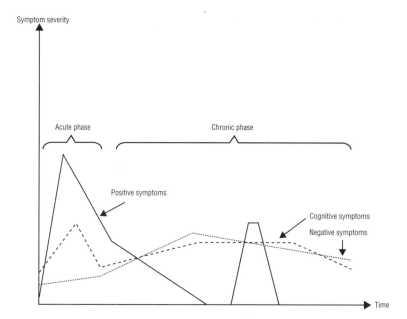

Figure 8: This diagram illustrates how the symptoms of schizophrenia may progress over time. As the course of the illness can vary, the diagram may not apply to individual cases.

of relapse include reduction or discontinuation of antipsychotic medication, alcohol and drug misuse, high expressed emotion, and continued stress. In some cases, the initial acute phase may be preceded by a so-called prodromal phase lasting for anything from days to years and consisting of subtle and non-specific abnormalities in thinking, feeling, and acting (see Chapter 4).

What causes the symptoms of schizophrenia?

According to the so-called dopamine hypothesis of schizophrenia, positive symptoms are produced by an *increase* in a chemical messenger called dopamine in a part of the brain called the mesolimbic tract (Figure 9). Evidence for this principally comes from a pair of observations,

1. Drugs that increase the level of dopamine in the mesolimbic tract, such as amphetamines and cannabis, can exacerbate the positive symptoms of schizophrenia or even induce a schizophrenia-like psychosis.

2. Antipsychotic medications that are effective in the treatment of the positive symptoms of schizophrenia block the effects of increased dopamine in the mesolimbic tract.

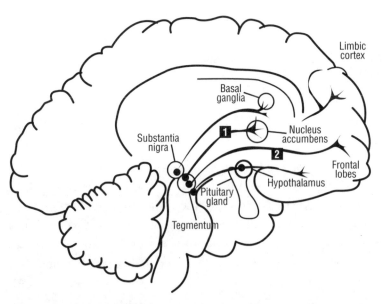

Figure 9: The dopamine hypothesis of schizophrenia. According to the dopamine hypothesis of schizophrenia, positive symptoms are thought to result from an increased level of dopamine in the mesolimbic tract (1), whereas negative symptoms are thought to result from a decreased level of dopamine in the mesocortical tract (2).

Negative symptoms on the other hand result from a *decrease* in dopamine in another part of the brain called the mesocortical tract (Figure 9). The principal evidence for this is that,

1. Drugs that increase the level of dopamine in the mesocortical tract can temporarily improve the negative symptoms of schizophrenia.
2. Older antipsychotic medications that can exacerbate the negative symptoms of schizophrenia block the effects of dopamine in the mesocortical tract.

The dopamine hypothesis has proved useful in providing a basic understanding of schizophrenia, but it says little about the actual cause of the changes in dopamine levels, and can by no means account for all the subtleties and complexities of the illness. Recent research has also implicated a number of other chemical messengers in the brain, for example, glutamate and serotonin, even though their precise roles are as yet unclear.

4

Diagnosis

The majority of medical conditions are defined by their cause ('aetiology') or by the bodily damage that they result in or from ('pathology'). For this reason, they are relatively easy to define and recognize. For example, malaria is caused by protozoan parasites of the genus *Plasmodium*, and cerebral infarction (that is, stroke) results from the obstruction of an artery in the brain. Unfortunately, schizophrenia cannot as yet be defined according to its aetiology or pathology, but only according to its clinical manifestations or symptoms. This means that a psychiatrist must base a diagnosis of schizophrenia solely on the patient's presentation, without any recourse to either blood tests (as in malaria) or brain scans (as in stroke).

When should help be sought?

There is strong scientific evidence that early detection and intervention improves outcomes of schizophrenia, for which reason many local mental healthcare teams provide a dedicated Early Intervention Service.

The first symptoms of schizophrenia can occur at any age, but they most commonly occur in the late teenage years or in early adulthood. These symptoms are often preceded by an insidious so-called prodromal phase lasting from days to months and consisting of subtle and non-specific abnormalities in thinking, feeling, and behaving (see Table 4).

Without the benefit of hindsight, the prodromal phase can be very difficult to recognize for what it is, especially as it so often occurs at an age when it can naturally be passed off as normal adolescent behaviour, relationship problems, depression, or substance misuse. It is therefore important for parents, relatives, and friends to 'trust their instincts' and to convince their loved one to seek medical advice from a general practitioner (GP) sooner rather than later. Depending on the nature, pattern, and severity of the symptoms, the GP may then decide to refer the person for a psychiatric opinion.

Table 4:   Prodromal symptoms of schizophrenia

Difficulty concentraing
Confusion
Decreased initiative and drive
Lack of energy
Flattened emotional response
Anxiety
Irritability
Depression
Sleeping late
Social isolation and withdrawal
Suspiciousness
Bizarre dress
Bizarre thoughts and thought patterns
Bizarre behaviour
Poor school performance
Poor self-care
Hearing voices

Case study

Valerie is a 23-year old anthropology student from Australia who shares a house with three other students on her course. Her housemates report that for the past six months Valerie has been behaving oddly, and that since the beginning of term four weeks ago she has not attended a single lecture. One month ago, she received a phone call informing her that her closest childhood friend, Chloe, had died in a motorbike accident. Since then,

Valerie has been locking herself in her room for increasing amounts of time, banging on the furniture, and apparently shouting to herself. Her housemates eventually persuaded her to see a doctor.

When Valerie arrived at the surgery, she was so agitated and distressed that she could not reply to most of the doctor's questions. The doctor was, however, able to make out that Valerie was hearing three or four male voices coming from outside her head: the voices were talking together about her, making fun of her, blaming her for her family's financial problems, and commenting on her thoughts and actions. According to Valerie, they were the voices of SAS paratroopers engaged by her parents to destroy her. Valerie said that they were trying to kill her by putting harmful thoughts, such as the thought of cutting her wrists, into her head.

Towards the end of the consultation, when the doctor stood up to hold the door open for her, Valerie screamed, 'I've seen your belt, they've sent you, they've sent you to distract me. I can't... I can't fight them any more!' and ran out of the room.

How is schizophrenia diagnosed?

If a person is suspected of having malaria, a blood sample can be taken and examined under a microscope for malarial parasites. Similarly, if a person is a suspected of having an abnormal rhythm of the heart, a heart tracing can be recorded so as to identify the abnormal rhythm. On the other hand, if a person is suspected of having schizophrenia, there are no laboratory or physical tests that can confirm the diagnosis. Instead, the psychiatrist must base the diagnosis on the person's symptoms, which must in turn meet certain agreed criteria listed in diagnostic manuals such as the International Classification of Diseases 10th Revision (ICD-10) and the Diagnostic and Statistical Manual of Mental Disorders 4th Revision (DSM-

IV). These criteria are validated by scientific research and, particularly in the case of ICD-10, by international consultation and consensus.

- First, the person must (in most cases) have at least one clear symptom that is characteristic of schizophrenia, such as delusions or hallucinations of voices.
- Second, these symptoms must have been present for at least one month, and signs of disturbance must have been present for at least six months.
- Third, these symptoms must be impacting on the person's level of social or occupational functioning.
- Fourth, other psychiatric and medical conditions that can present like schizophrenia must have been excluded (see Table 5 for a list of these conditions).

Table 5: Conditions that can present like schizophrenia

Psychiatric conditions
Drug use – for example, cannabis, amphetamines, cocaine and LSD
Severe depression with psychotic symptoms
Bipolar affective disorder: severe depression with psychotic symptoms or mania (elevated mood) with psychotic symptoms
Schizoaffective disorder: more or less equally prominent symptoms of both schizophrenia and mood disorder (depression or mania)
Other psychotic disorders such as brief psychotic disorder, a condition which resembles schizophrenia but is relatively short-lived
Personality disorder

Medical conditions
Temporal lobe epilepsy
Head injury
Dementia
Stroke
Brain tumour
Infectious diseases affecting the brain
Endocrine disorders such as Cushing's syndrome
Metabolic disorders such as vitamin B12 deficiency

How long does it take to make a diagnosis of schizophrenia?

Once schizophrenia is suspected, the psychiatrist sets about excluding psychiatric and medical conditions that can present similarly by obtaining a clear and detailed picture of the person's symptoms and personal background, often over a protracted period of time. During this time, he or she may also conduct a full physical examination, obtain blood and urine samples, and arrange for a brain scan such as a CT or MRI scan. In some cases, he or she may arrange for a second psychiatrist or other specialist (such as a neurologist or endocrinologist) to provide a second opinion. Only after the psychiatrist has confidently ruled out other psychiatric and medical conditions can a firm diagnosis of schizophrenia be made.

After developing the first symptoms of schizophrenia, it can take several weeks before a confident diagnosis of schizophrenia can be made (although this does not mean that appropriate treatment for severe and distressing or disabling symptoms cannot be started). This limbo period can be one of the most difficult times for the schizophrenia sufferer and his or her relatives.

If schizophrenia cannot be diagnosed in its prodromal phase, how is early intervention possible?

Schizophrenia is diagnosed from its positive, cognitive, and negative symptoms, which means that the illness cannot be diagnosed in its early, prodromal phase when these symptoms are still lacking or poorly formed. However, this does not mean that the illness cannot be strongly suspected or that appropriate treatment cannot be considered. The role of early detection and intervention in improving outcomes cannot be overemphasized.

5

Coping with a diagnosis of schizophrenia

A diagnosis of schizophrenia is difficult to accept, both for the person diagnosed and for his or her relatives. Like heart disease or diabetes, schizophrenia is a serious and potentially debilitating illness. But unlike heart disease or diabetes—or even other psychiatric conditions such as depression or panic attacks— schizophrenia is poorly understood and heavily stigmatized by the general public. This is in no small part due to sensationalist reporting in the media of violent acts committed by a small number of schizophrenia sufferers. The reality is of course that schizophrenia is a common illness that can be treated effectively and that only rarely results in people becoming aggressive or dangerous.

Given this state of affairs, it can be no surprise that some people with a fresh diagnosis of schizophrenia decide (or are persuaded) to consult a second or third psychiatrist, often at great expense, in the hope of having their diagnosis changed or reversed. Others might simply deny the diagnosis, and instead refer to the illness as 'depression', 'bipolar affective disorder', or some other mental disorder. Yet others might tell people that they are in hospital because they have a brain tumour or because they are undertaking a drug rehabilitation programme. Some, especially those suffering from prominent positive symptoms such as delusions and hallucinations, may altogether deny that they are ill—not only because they can't bear the stigma attached to a label of schizophrenia, but also because their delusions and hallucinations seem perfectly real to them, and, in some cases, prevent them from trusting or believing other people. For example, a person who is suffering from the delusion of being persecuted by the secret services may believe that his psychiatrist is in fact a special agent in disguise, and therefore that he is being lied to.

In contrast, some people experience a profound sense of relief at receiving a diagnosis of schizophrenia because it enables them to get the help that they need, and to make the fastest and most complete recovery possible.

Unlike illness such as heart disease or diabetes, schizophrenia tends to strike in the prime of life when people are likely to be full of plans and hopes for the future. In some cases, they may feel under intense pressure to succeed and be successful. Many people with a fresh diagnosis of schizophrenia feel that all their dreams have been shattered and that they have betrayed themselves and all those around them. Mixed feelings of loss, hopelessness, and guilt may give rise to a depressive illness, and, in some cases, even to thoughts of self-harm and suicide. In such cases, it is important to bear in mind that increasing numbers of schizophrenia sufferers do make a full recovery, and that many others are able to lead productive and fulfilling lives. Indeed, some schizophrenia sufferers, such as John Nash, the Nobel laureate in economics, and Tom Harrell, the jazz trumpeter, have even gone on to make unique and important contributions to society. You can make the future yours again, just as you are doing by making the effort to read this book.

Here is Robert Bayley again, this time writing about his experience of coping with schizophrenia,

Despite the onslaught, there remains fertile ground. Areas where creativity can thrive. Physical discipline can also be applied, to aid the altering of the brain's chemistry. And beneath all this, the intrinsic will to survive. To remain positive, when all around

is coated with despair. For I believe that I can advance, I can develop strategies that will lead me into tomorrows. I will not be beaten. I will continue to create, make something beautiful from the extremes of madness. One day I will shout from the rooftops, all torment removed.

Do remember: you are not to blame for your illness, and you must not think that you have done anything to 'deserve' it. Do not let your parents blame themselves for your illness either. Just like anybody else, people with schizophrenia can have good parents, bad parents, or absent parents. Far from being to blame, parents are often their child's most valuable source of structure and support, and their greatest hope for a safe and permanent

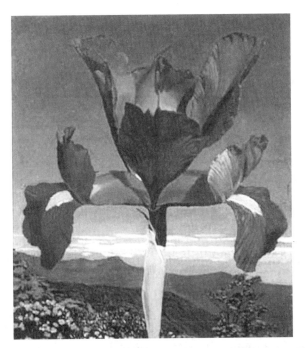

Figure 10:   'Blue Iris' by schizophrenia sufferer Bryan Charnley. The petals are like three flags: one for hope, one for faith, and one for courage (SANE/Bryan Charnley).

recovery. Schizophrenia is a common illness that is in large part genetically determined. It is not helpful to think of it as anybody's fault.

Many schizophrenia sufferers find it difficult to accept that they are mentally ill, and, as a result, can be reluctant to help themselves or accept help from others. Schizophrenia is a serious illness and leaving it untreated can have grave consequences for your short-term and long-term mental and physical health. The fear, isolation, and difficulty in carrying out even the simplest of tasks can lead to a vicious cycle of neglect, depression, and alcohol and drug use. By accepting your psychiatrist's diagnosis, talking and reading about it, and seeking the help that you need, you are taking personal control over your illness and giving yourself the best chances of a long-term recovery. Remember that you are not alone, and that many people have once been in a similar situation. Meeting and exchanging with these people can provide you with much-needed information and support, and help to alleviate any feelings of fear or isolation that you may have.

Will I get better?

Hopefully, yes. Although there is no miracle cure, schizophrenia can be successfully treated:

- About 1 in 4 people recover completely within a five-year period.
- About 2 in 4 people get better but suffer from occasional relapses. The number and frequency of relapses often depends on the quality of long-term care and support and on continued compliance with antipsychotic medication.
- About 1 in 4 people continue to suffer from symptoms on a permanent or almost permanent basis. Yet even in these cases, treatment and support can do much to alleviate symptoms and improve personal functioning and quality of life.

A person's individual chances of getting better are difficult to predict, but certain factors related to his or her personal circumstances and to the severity of the illness can act as 'positive prognostic factors'—factors that make a positive outcome more likely. Positive and negative prognostic factors in schizophrenia are listed in Table 6. Some prognostic factors, such as a person's gender or family history, obviously cannot be changed; but many others, such as receiving early treatment and remaining on antipsychotic medication, are entirely within your personal control.

Table 6: Positive and negative prognostic factors in schizophrenia

Positive prognostic factors	Negative prognostic factors
Acute (rapid) onset	Insidious (gradual) onset
Onset at an older age	Onset at an earlier age
Clear precipitating factors such as life events	Absence of clear precipitating factors
Florid positive symptoms and associated mood disorder	Prominent negative symptoms
Female sex	Male sex
No family history	Strong family history
No alcohol or drug misuse	Frequent alcohol and drug misuse
Good occupational and social functioning before the start of the illness	Poor occupational and social functioning before the start of the illness
Good social support and stimulation	Poor social support and stimulation
Being married or in a partnership	Being single, separated or divorced
Receiving early treatment	Delaying treatment
Making a good response to treatment	Making a poor response to treatment
Remaining on antipsychotic medication	Stopping antipsychotic medication or not taking it regularly

Life expectancy in schizophrenia varies quite a lot, and in large part depends upon the severity and, especially, the duration of the illness. Overall, the life expectancy of people with schizophrenia is reduced by about 8–10 years compared to average, but this gap is closing thanks to more effective treatments and interventions together with higher standards of physical care. Perhaps surprisingly, cardiovascular diseases are the leading cause of death in schizophrenia sufferers. One of the greatest contributors to cardiovascular diseases in schizophrenia sufferers is smoking, so stopping smoking—together with diet control and regular exercise—can do much to increase life expectancy (see Chapter 8). Other important causes of death in schizophrenia sufferers are accidents, drug overdoses, and, in a small but significant minority, self-harm and suicide.

The suicide rate in schizophrenia sufferers is of the order of 5 per cent, although the rate of attempted suicide (an attempt at suicide that is ultimately unsuccessful) and self-harm is significantly higher. Factors that increase the likelihood of suicide in schizophrenia include being male, being young, being unmarried, lacking social support, scoring above average on IQ tests, having high ambitions and expectations, being early in the course of the illness, maintaining or developing good insight into the illness, and being recently discharged from a psychiatric hospital.

Depression

If relatives suspect that their loved one is suffering from symptoms of depression, they should bring this to the attention of a member of the mental healthcare team so that the symptoms can be addressed. Sometimes it can be difficult to tell apart the symptoms of depression from the negative symptoms of schizophrenia or from the side effects of antipsychotic medication. However, depression is common in schizophrenia sufferers and it is best to have a high index of suspicion and to seek advice sooner rather than later. The symptoms of depression are listed in Table 7. See Chapter 8 for some simple advice on beating depression.

Table 7:   Symptoms of depression

Core features of depression
Sadness
Lack of interest and enjoyment
Feeling tired easily

Psychological features of depression
Poor concentration
Poor motivation and energy
Poor self-esteem and self-confidence
Feelings of guilt
Pessimistic outlook

Biological features of depression
Sleep disturbance – for example, waking up very early in the morning
Loss of appetite and/or weight loss
Loss of libido
Retardation (slowing down) of speech and movements

What does depression feel like?

William Styron, author of *Sophie's Choice* and other novels, wrote a book called *Darkness Visible* about his personal struggle with depression. Here is an extract,

> *In depression this faith in deliverance, in ultimate restoration, is absent. The pain is unrelenting, and what makes the condition intolerable is the foreknowledge that no remedy will come—not in a day, an hour, a month, or a minute. If there is mild relief, one knows that it is only temporary; more pain will follow. It is hopelessness even more than pain that crushes the soul. So the decision-making of daily life involves not, as in normal affairs, shifting from one annoying situation to another less annoying— or from discomfort to relative comfort, or from boredom to activity—but moving from pain to pain. One does not abandon, even briefly, one's bed of nails, but is attached to it wherever one goes.*

Rehabilitation

A minority of people with schizophrenia, especially those suffering from prominent negative symptoms, may in due course benefit from a period of rehabilitation, the aim of which is to bring them to their highest possible level of functioning. Areas that are considered during rehabilitation include activities of daily living (for example, activities around personal hygiene, meal preparation, and shopping), occupational activities, leisure activities, and social skills. Sheltered employment programmes that use the place-and-train vocational model can significantly increase a schizophrenia sufferer's likelihood of one day gaining competitive employment.

Despite a period of rehabilitation, a small number of schizophrenia sufferers may be unable to live independently, and may therefore require some form of supported accommodation. Supported accommodation is often found is a sheltered home or group home—a house shared by several schizophrenia sufferers and supported by a group homes organization.

6

Mental healthcare services

Some 40 or 50 years ago, many if not most people with a first episode of schizophrenia would have been admitted to a psychiatric hospital for assessment and treatment, and some may have remained as inpatients for an indefinitely long period of time. In the 1950s and 1960s, this institutional model of psychiatric care came under heavy criticism for isolating and institutionalizing schizophrenia sufferers and, in so doing, reinforcing the stigma attached to them and to their illness. This led to a trend of removing schizophrenia sufferers from psychiatric hospitals in the hope of re-integrating them into the community. This trend, greatly facilitated by the advent of the first antipsychotic drugs in the 1950s and 1960s, continued throughout the 1970s and 1980s.

In the 1980s, the community care approach came under attack after a series of headline-grabbing killings by schizophrenia sufferers. Although acts of violence by schizophrenia sufferers are rare, they are often sensationally reported in the media, creating the false impression that schizophrenia-sufferers are an especially dangerous group of people. The truth is, of course, very different: schizophrenia sufferers are sensitive and vulnerable, and in great need of care and understanding. A small minority may pose a risk, but this risk is far more often to themselves than to others.

The public outcry surrounding the community care approach prompted a government inquiry that culminated in the Community Care Act of 1990, a major piece of legislation that is at the origins of the present, more 'fail-safe' model of community care. One major difference is that, prior to discharge from a psychiatric hospital, every person should have an agreed care plan for continued treatment and support in the community.

The advantages of community care are clear. By shifting the emphasis from a person's mental illness to his or her strengths and life aspirations, community care promotes independence and self-reliance while discouraging isolation and institutionalization and reducing stigma and stigmatization. That having been said, a lack of mental healthcare staff and resources can in some cases shift the burden of care onto informal carers such as relatives and friends, and make it especially difficult to care for those most in need, namely, the isolated and the homeless. The advantages and disadvantages of community care are listed in Table 8.

Table 8:   Advantages and disadvantages of community care

Advantages	Disadvantages or problems
By focusing on strengths and life aspirations rather than on psychiatric problems, promotes independence and self-reliance	Lack of staff and resources can place a heavy burden on carers
Discourages isolation and institutionalization	Makes it difficult to provide care for those most in need, such as the homeless
Promotes relapse prevention	Results in a shortage of hospital beds as scarce resources are diverted to community services
Reduces the stigma of mental illness	
Originally thought to be cheaper than in-patient care, but this notion has more recently been challenged	In some cases results in the mentally ill becoming homeless, or being housed in the prison service rather than in hospitals
	Poses a (possibly mainly perceived) threat to the safety of the person and of the community

One Flew Over the Cuckoo's Nest

Vintery, mintery, cutery, corn,
Apple seed and apple thorn;
Wire, briar, limber, lock,
Three geese in a flock.
One flew east, And one flew west,
And one flew over the cuckoo's nest.
         —Popular nursery rhyme

The film *One Flew over the Cuckoo's Nest*, adapted from Ken Kasey's popular 1962 novel of the same name, was directed by Milos Forman and starred Jack Nicholson as the spirited RP McMurphy ('Mac') and Louise Fletcher as the chilly but softly-spoken Nurse Ratched. When Mac arrives at the state mental hospital in Oregon, he challenges the stultifying routine and bureaucratic authoritarianism personified by Nurse Ratched, and pays the price by being drugged, electroshocked, and—ultimately—lobotomized. Nominated for 9 Academy Awards, the film is not only a (belated and contentious) criticism of the institutional model of psychiatric care, but also a metaphor of total institutions—that is, institutions that repress individuality to create a compliant society. It is such criticism of the institutional model of psychiatric care that, in the UK and other countries, led to the development of community care.

The organization of mental healthcare services

General Practice and A&E

If a person is suffering from symptoms similar to those seen in schizophrenia, the first port of call is usually the family doctor or general practitioner (GP). If the GP forms an opinion that the person is suffering from schizophrenia or another psychotic illness, then he or she is likely to refer the person to specialist mental health services—either to a local Community

Mental Health Team (CMHT) or, in an emergency, to the Crisis Resolution and Home Treatment Team (CRHT).

A minority of people with symptoms of schizophrenia first present to Accident and Emergency (A&E) rather than to their GP. In this case, they are usually screened by a casualty doctor, and then referred for assessment by a psychiatrist. Again—if the psychiatrist forms an opinion that the person is suffering from schizophrenia or another psychotic illness, then he or she is most likely to refer the person to a local CMHT or, in an emergency, to the CRHT. The organization of mental healthcare services is represented in Figure 11.

Community Mental Health Team, Early Intervention Service, and Assertive Outreach Team

These three entities are listed together as they often operate from the same community base. The Community Mental Health Team (CMHT) is at the centre of mental healthcare provision. It is a multidisciplinary team led by a consultant psychiatrist and operating from a team base close to the patients that it serves. Community psychiatric nurses (CPNs) and social workers are key members of the CMHT, and often take a lead in implementing and coordinating a person's care and treatment plan, as well as in monitoring his or her progress in the community. Other important members of the CMHT include psychiatrists, clinical psychologists, occupational therapists, pharmacists, and administrative staff (Table 9). If a person is referred to a CMHT, he or she usually undergoes an initial assessment by a psychiatrist, sometimes in the presence of another member of the team such as a CPN or social worker. This modern, multidisciplinary approach ensures that the different parts of the person's life can be understood—and addressed—from a number of different angles.

Some people are reluctant to seek help and treatment, and as a consequence appear at the CMHT only at times of crisis.

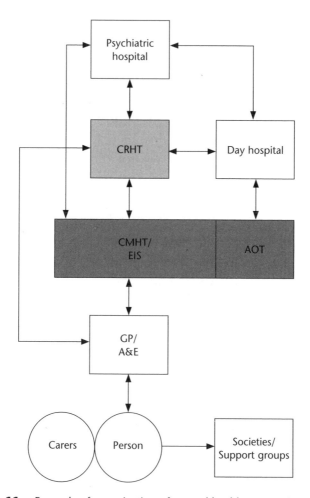

Figure 11:   Example of organization of mental healthcare services (local services may differ). Note that mental healthcare services are organized so as to facilitate community care and avoid unnecessary hospital admissions. All terms used in this figure are explained in the chapter. CRHT, Crisis Resolution and Home Treatment Team; CMHT, Community Mental Health Team; EIS, Early Intervention Service; AOT or AORT, Assertive Outreach Team; GP, general practitioner; A&E, Accident and Emergency department.

Paradoxically, these so-called revolving door patients often have the greatest mental health and social problems. The responsibility for their care is sometimes delegated to the Assertive Outreach Team (AOT), a specialized multidisciplinary that aims to engage them in treatment and support them in their daily activities.

Like the AOT, the Early Intervention Service (EIS) may also operate from the CMHT base. Its role is specifically to improve the short- and long-term outcomes of schizophrenia and other psychotic illnesses by a three-pronged approach involving (1) preventative measures, (2) earlier detection of untreated cases, and (3) intensive treatment and support in the early stages of the illness.

Table 9:   Key members of the Community Mental Health Team

Psychiatrist	The psychiatrist is a medical doctor who specializes in diagnosing and treating mental illnesses, such as schizophrenia, bipolar affective disorder, depressive disorders and anxiety disorders. The psychiatrist takes a leading role in diagnosing mental illness and formulating a treatment plan
Community psychiatric nurse (CPN)	The CPN is the member of the team that the schizophrenia sufferer is likely to come into contact with most often. The CPN usually visits him or her to monitor his or her progress and facilitate his or her treatment plan
Social worker	Sometimes a schizophrenia sufferer may be allocated a social worker as well as or instead of a CPN, in which case the social worker fulfils a role similar to that of the CPN. The social worker can also help to sort out housing and benefits and to ensure that the schizophrenia sufferer makes the most of any services and facilities that are available
Clinical psychologist	'Psychologist' is often confused with 'psychiatrist'. Whereas a psychiatrist is a medical doctor specializing in the diagnosis and treatment of mental illness, a psychologist has expertise of human experience and behaviour. A psychologist may spend time listening to and trying to understand the schizophrenia sufferer and his or her carers. A psychologist may also carry out talking therapies such as cognitive-behavioural therapy or family therapy, which are discussed in greater detail in Chapter 8

Occupational therapist	The role of the occupational therapist is to help the schizophrenia sufferer to maintain his or her skills as well as to develop new ones. This not only helps him or her to get back to work, but also keeps him or her engaged and motivated. Unfortunately, owing to limited resources, many schizophrenia sufferers are not allocated an occupational therapist
Pharmacist	Schizophrenia sufferers who also have a physical illness or who are pregnant or breast-feeding may find it particularly useful to speak to a pharmacist, who can help with information about medication
Administrative staff	Administrative staff are responsible for arranging appointments and serve as a crucial point of contact for both schizophrenia sufferers and their carers and other members of the team

Other forms of support that are available but that do not form part of the CMHT include support groups, telephone helplines (see Useful addresses) and the Citizens Advice Bureau.

Crisis Resolution and Home Treatment Team

The Crisis Resolution and Home Treatment Team (CRHT), or 'crisis team' for short, is a 24-hours-a-day, 365-days-a-year multidisciplinary team that acts as a gatekeeper to a variety of psychiatric services, including admission to a psychiatric hospital. People with acute mental health problems are referred to the CRHT from a variety of places and agencies, most commonly GPs, A&E, and CMHTs. A member of the team (often a community psychiatric nurse) promptly assesses the person in conjunction with a psychiatrist to determine if hospital admission can be avoided through the provision of short-term intensive home care. If so, the CRHT arranges for a member of the team to visit the person's home up to three times a day, gradually decreasing the frequency of visits as he or she gets better. Other than simply providing support, the CRHT can also assist in implementing a care and treatment plan and in monitoring progress. If the person has already been admitted to hospital, the CRHT can be involved in expediting and/or facilitating his or her discharge back into the community. The key features of the CRHT are summarized in Table 10.

Table 10:   Key features of the Crisis Resolution and Home Treatment Team

Gatekeeper to psychiatric services, including admission to a psychiatric hospital

Prompt assessment of patients in a crisis

Intensive, community-based, round-the-clock support in the early stages of the crisis

Continued involvement until the crisis has resolved

Work to prevent similar crises from occurring again

Partnership with the schizophrenia sufferer and his or her relatives and carers

Psychiatric Hospital and Day Hospital

Under the current model of community care, the vast majority of people with a first or subsequent episode of schizophrenia are treated in the community: if a person is admitted to hospital, then this is usually because care in the community is not a viable option. Possible reasons for admission to a psychiatric hospital are summarized in Table 11.

Table 11:   Possible reasons for admission to a psychiatric hospital

Safety of the schizophrenia sufferer, his or her carers and the general public

Management of acute exacerbations (e.g. severe psychotic symptoms)

Management of physical complications (e.g. accidents)

Stabilization of medication

Establishment of a diagnosis

Alternative to community care if the schizophrenia sufferer lacks adequate support in the community

Respite for the carer

Of the small number of people with schizophrenia who need to be admitted to a psychiatric hospital, a majority are admitted on a voluntary, informal basis. People admitted on a voluntary basis are happy to accept the advice of their psychiatrist or carers, and/or are frightened of their symptoms and feel that the psychiatric hospital is a relatively safe place to be. In some cases, attendance at a day hospital during office hours only (from around 9am to around 5pm) may provide people with a more tolerable alternative to hospital admission.

A minority of people with schizophrenia who need to be admitted to a psychiatric hospital refuse to be admitted, usually because they lack insight into their mental illness. In many countries—and certainly in all industrialized countries—there are special legal provisions to protect such people from the potential consequences of their illness. In England and Wales,

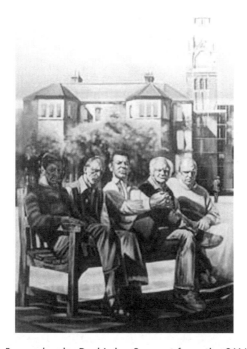

Figure 12:   *Barmy days* by Paul Lake. Support from the SANE Arts Grant Scheme helped Paul to achieve his ambition to become a successful artist. *Barmy days* is a portrait of himself and some friends at the Brookwood Psychiatric Hospital. 'I wanted to show the positive side of the mental hospital and the way it allowed us the time and space to accept our illness.'

the Mental Health Act is the principal legal document governing not only the compulsory detention of people in a psychiatric hospital, but also their treatment, discharge from hospital, and aftercare. The equivalent legislation in Scotland is the Mental Health (Care and Treatment) Act 2003, and in Northern Ireland the Mental Health (Northern Ireland) Order 1986. A person admitted to hospital under one of these Acts does not lose all rights to make decisions about his or her future; soon after being admitted to hospital, the person has his or her rights explained by a member of staff, and can also ask for this information to be provided in writing. In the United States, the requirements and procedures for compulsory detention vary from state to state, but are broadly in line with those in the countries of the United Kingdom.

The Mental Health Act

People with a mental disorder as defined by the Mental Health Act can be detained under the Act in the interests of their health or safety and/or in the interests of protecting the general public. To minimize the potential for abuse, the Act specifically excludes dependence on alcohol or drugs as mental disorders.

Section 2

Two of the most common 'Sections' of the Mental Health Act that are used to admit people with a mental disorder to a psychiatric hospital are the so-called Sections 2 and 3. Section 2 allows for an admission for assessment and treatment that can last for up to 28 days. An application for a section 2 is usually made by an Approved Mental Health Professional (AMHP) with special training in mental health and recommended by two doctors, one of whom must have special experience in the diagnosis and treatment of mental disorders. Under a Section 2, treatment can be given, but only if it is aimed at treating the mental disorder or conditions directly resulting from the mental disorder. A Section 2 can be 'discharged' or revoked at any time by the Responsible Clinician (usually the consultant psychiatrist in charge), by the hospital managers, or by the person's nearest relative. Moreover, a person detained under a Section 2 can appeal against the Section in which case his or her appeal is considered by a specially constituted tribunal. A solicitor represents the person to the tribunal and helps him or her to make a case in favour of discharge. The tribunal is by nature adversarial, and it falls upon members of the detained person's care team to argue the case for continued detention. This can be quite trying for everyone involved, and can at times undermine the person's trust in his or her care team. Section 2 is broadly equivalent to Section 26 of the Mental Health (Care and Treatment) (Scotland) Act 2003, except that Section 26 cannot be used to admit the person to hospital. Instead, Section 26 tags onto Section 24 (Emergency Admission to Hospital) or Section 25 (Detention of Patients Already in Hospital).

Section 3

A person can be detained under a Section 3 after a conclusive period of assessment under a Section 2. Alternatively, the person can be detained directly under a Section 3 if his or her diagnosis has already been established by the care team and is not in reasonable doubt. Section 3 corresponds to an admission for treatment and lasts for up to 6 months. As for a Section 2, it is usually applied for by an AMHP with special training in mental health and approved by two doctors, one of whom must have special experience in the diagnosis and treatment of mental disorders. Treatment under a Section 3 can only be given if it is aimed at treating the mental disorder or conditions directly resulting from the mental disorder. After the first 3 months, any treatment requires either the consent of the person being treated or the recommendation of a second doctor. A Section 3 can be discharged at any time by the Responsible Clinician (usually the consultant psychiatrist in charge), the hospital managers, or the person's nearest relative. Moreover, a person detained under a Section 3 can appeal against the Section in which case his or her appeal is considered by a specially constituted tribunal, as detailed above. If the person still needs to be detained after the 6 months have elapsed, the Section 3 can be renewed for further periods. Section 3 is broadly similar to Section 18 of the Mental Health (Care and Treatment) (Scotland) Act 2003.

Other commonly used Sections of the Mental Health Act

The other Sections of the Mental Health Act that you might come across are Sections 135 and 136, the so-called 'police Sections', and Section 5(2), the doctor's emergency holding order.

Section 135 authorizes removal by the police of a person from his or her premises to a place of safety, and is valid for 72 hours. Section 136 authorizes removal by the police of a person from a public place (such as a park or a street) to a place of safety, and is also valid for 72 hours.

A person who has already been admitted to hospital and who needs to be prevented from leaving on the grounds of mental disorder can be placed under a Section 5(2) by the doctor in charge of the patient's care or by a nominated deputy such as the doctor on call. A Section 5(2) is valid for 72 hours; it expires as soon as the patient has been formally assessed under the Mental Health Act and either released or detained (usually under a Section 2 or 3). Unlike a Section 2 or 3, a Section 5(2) does not authorize treatment of the mental disorder.

Aftercare

If a person has been detained under Section 3 of the Mental Health Act, he or she is automatically placed under a Section 117 at the time of discharge from Section 3. Section 117 corresponds to 'aftercare' and places a duty on the local health authority and local social services authority to provide the person with a care package aimed at rehabilitation and relapse prevention. Although the person is under no obligation to accept aftercare, in some cases he or she may also be placed under 'Supervised Community Treatment' or 'Guardianship' to ensure that he or she receives aftercare. Under Supervised Community Treatment, the person is made subject to certain conditions; if these conditions are not met, then he or she can be recalled into hospital.

The Care Programme Approach

The longer-term care and treatment of people accepted into specialist mental healthcare services is usually planned at one or several Care Programme Approach (CPA) meetings attended by both the schizophrenia sufferer and his or her carers. These meetings are useful to establish the context of the schizophrenia sufferer's illness; evaluate his or her current personal circumstances; assess his or her medical, psychological, and social needs; and formulate a detailed care and treatment plan to ensure that these needs are met. As well as ensuring that the schizophrenia sufferer takes his or her medication and is regularly seen by a psychiatrist or CPN, this care and treatment plan may involve a number of psychological or social interventions such as attendance at self-help groups, carer education and support, home help, cognitive-behavioural therapy, and rehabilitation. A care co-ordinator, most often a CPN or social worker, is appointed to ensure that the care and treatment plan is implemented and revised in light of changing circumstances. The people who generally attend CPA meetings are listed in Table 12. At the outcome of a CPA meeting, the schizophrenia sufferer should feel that his or her needs, circumstances, and preferences have been fully understood, and that the care plan that he or she has helped to formulate reflects these in as far as possible.

Table 12:   People who may attend Care Programme Approach meetings

The schizophrenia sufferer

Relatives or advocates of the schizophrenia sufferer

The Responsible Medical Officer (usually a consultant psychiatrist)

Other psychiatrists

The GP

The care co-ordinator (most often a community psychiatric nurse or social worker)

A community psychiatric nurse

A social worker

An occupational therapist

A worker from the schizophrenia sufferer's residential home, day placement or home

7

Antipsychotic medication

Although there is no miracle cure for schizophrenia, the illness can be successfully treated, and three out of four schizophrenia sufferers can expect either to make a full recovery or to improve significantly. Antipsychotic medication is usually the mainstay of treatment, but psychosocial interventions such as patient and family education, self-help groups, illness self-management, social and vocational skills training, and cognitive-behavioural therapy can all play an important role in reducing symptoms, preventing relapse and re-hospitalization, and helping you to regain control over your life. Psychosocial treatments are discussed in Chapter 8.

How do antipsychotics work?

You may recall from Chapter 3 that, according to the dopamine hypothesis, the positive symptoms of schizophrenia (delusions and hallucinations) result from an increased level of the chemical messenger dopamine in a part of the brain called the mesolimbic tract. Antipsychotics are effective in the treatment of positive symptoms because they block the action of dopamine in the mesolimbic tract.

How effective are antipsychotics?

Antipsychotic medication is effective in controlling positive symptoms in about 70–80 per cent of schizophrenia sufferers, although it can be several days before the effects are fully felt. Until then, the schizophrenia sufferer may benefit from taking a sedative such as lorazepam if he or she is highly distressed or agitated. In some cases, several antipsychotics may need to be trialled before one that is both effective and without troublesome side effects can be found. Unfortunately, antipsychotics have relatively little effect on the cognitive and negative symptoms of schizophrenia.

Are antipsychotics always needed?

Scientific research has conclusively demonstrated that long-term antipsychotic treatment reduces rates of relapse and re-hospitalization in a substantial number of schizophrenia sufferers. Although non-pharmacological, psychosocial treatments have an important role to play in the management of schizophrenia (see Chapter 8), the current consensus is that an antipsychotic is always needed.

Many people quite understandably do not like taking too much medication, most often because they are frightened of becoming addicted to pills or reluctant to put up with undesirable side effects. Like all medication, antipsychotic medication can have side effects; however, it is not in any sense addictive. The effective management of schizophrenia involves balancing the risks and benefits of treatment with antipsychotic medication and reassessing that balance in light of changing circumstances. It is important to remember that not all people on antipsychotic medication suffer from side effects, and that many side effects are only mild or temporary or easily addressed by simple lifestyle changes. If you decide to reduce or come off your antipsychotic medication, do make sure to discuss and agree this with your mental healthcare team first. You should not stop your medication at once, but decrease it gradually over a long period of time. During this time, your mental state should be monitored at frequent and regular intervals so that your medication can be stepped up at the first sign of a potential relapse.

Which antipsychotic is the best?

Current treatment guidelines for the treatment of schizophrenia recommend starting on one of the more recent (so-called 'atypical') antipsychotics, which, compared with the older (so-called 'typical') antipsychotics, are less likely to produce certain disturbing side effects called extrapyramidal side effects (see later). Atypical antipsychotics may also have greater efficacy against cognitive and negative symptoms than the older typical antipsychotics. That having been said, many schizophrenia sufferers who have been on antipsychotic medication for many years prefer to remain on an older typical antipsychotic than to risk the changeover to an atypical antipsychotic.

There are several atypical antipsychotics, with risperidone, olanzapine, and quetiapine being among the most commonly prescribed. While these antipsychotics are on balance similarly effective, they do have slightly different side effects. In addition, some antipsychotics come in different forms that may be easier to take. For example, some antipsychotics come in liquid form or as an oral dispersible tablet (ODT) that dissolves in the mouth. The various factors involved in choosing an antipsychotic medication are listed in Table 13.

Table 13:   Principal factors involved in choosing an antipsychotic

Initially
Particular side effect(s) that the schizophrenia sufferer is keen to avoid
Any previous side effects that he or she found to be unacceptable
Difficulties that he or she anticipates in taking the antipsychotic in standard tablet form

Later in the course of treatment
Effectiveness of antipsychotic in controlling the schizophrenia sufferer's symptoms
Current side effects that he or she finds to be unacceptable
Difficulties that he or she has in taking the antipsychotic in standard table form

As aforementioned, some people might need to trial several antipsychotics before finding the one that suits them best. This period of 'trial and error' is particularly difficult because the antipsychotics are either not working or producing intolerable side effects. Although sharing experiences can be useful, it is important not to be overly influenced by other people's individual experiences with various antipsychotics. Every person is unique, and there is no one antipsychotic that best suits all.

What questions should I ask my doctor before starting on an antipsychotic?

Questions that you should ask your doctor before starting on an antipsychotic include:

- How will it help me?
- How should I take it?
- How long will it take to work?
- How long do I need to take it for?
- What side effects am I risking?
- Can I do anything to avoid or reduce these side effects?
- Whom should I get in touch with if there is a problem?

What are the side-effects of antipsychotic medication?

Antipsychotics are effective in the treatment of positive symptoms because they block the effects of dopamine in the mesolimbic tract. Unfortunately they can also block the effects of dopamine in other brain tracts, resulting in a number of unpleasant side effects.

- If an antipsychotic blocks the effects of dopamine in the nigrostriatal tract (see Figure 13), this can lead to extra-pyramidal side effects, that is, to disturbances of voluntary muscle function. The four recognized types of extrapyramidal side effects are listed in Table 14.

- If an antipsychotic blocks the effects of dopamine in the tuberoinfundibular tract, this can lead to an increase in the hormone prolactin (a state called 'hyperprolactinaemia'), which can result in a loss of libido and also, in men, erectile dysfunction.

- If an antipsychotic blocks the effects of dopamine in the mesocortical tract, this can exacerbate the negative symptoms of schizophrenia, which, as you might recall from Chapter 3, are caused by a decrease of dopamine in this tract.

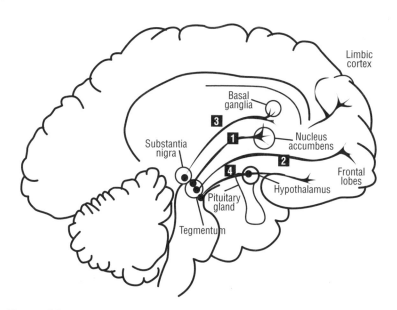

Figure 13: Dopamine projections in the brain, showing the mesolimbic tract (1) (positive symptoms of schizophrenia), the mesocortical tract (2) (negative symptoms of schizophrenia), the nigrostriatal tract (3) (extrapyramidal side effects of antipsychotic medication), and the tuberoinfundibular tract (4) (sexual side effects of antipsychotic medication).

Table 14:　Extrapyramidal side effects of antipsychotics

Acute dystonias	Acute dystonias involve painful contractions of a muscle or muscle group, most commonly in the neck, eyes and trunk. They are usually easily recognized and successfully treated with anticholinergic medication such as procyclidine, orphenadrine or benzhexol
Akathisia	Akathisia involves a distressing feeling of inner restlessness, manifested by fidgety leg movements, shuffling of the feet and pacing. As akathisia is readily confused with the positive symptoms of schizophrenia, it can sometimes be difficult to recognize. Treatment usually involves reducing the dose of antipsychotic or changing to another antipsychotic
Parkinson-like symptoms	Parkinson-like symptoms principally involve three features: tremor, muscular rigidity and difficulty starting movements. Parkinson-like symptoms may respond to anticholinergic medication, although it is often preferable to reduce the dose of antipsychotic or change to another antipsychotic
Tardive dyskinesia	Tardive dyskinesia usually occurs after several months or years of antipsychotic treatment and is often irreversible. It involves involuntary, repetitive, purposeless movements of the tongue, lips, face, trunk and extremities. The movements may be generalized or affect only certain muscle groups, typically the muscles around the mouth. There is no consistently beneficial treatment, and the condition may be exacerbated by anticholinergic medication. Since the advent of atypical antipsychotics, tardive dyskinesia has become considerably less common

Antipsychotics can also interfere with other neurotransmitters in the brain, which may potentially produce further side effects. An important and common side effect is sedation, although some degree of sedation can actually be beneficial in people with distressing positive symptoms. Another important and common side effect is weight gain, which can place people at long-term risk of heart disease and diabetes. For these reasons, it is important to have your physical health monitored, develop and maintain healthy eating habits, take regular exercise, and avoid smoking. Other common side effects of antipsychotics include orthostatic hypotension (dizziness upon sitting up and standing) and so-called anticholinergic side effects such as dry mouth, blurred vision, and constipation. Any side effects that have not been mentioned are comparatively uncommon and may not be caused by every antipsychotic.

Because there are such a large number of antipsychotics to choose from, people need not expect to suffer from unacceptable side effects. If you feel that you are suffering from intolerable side effects, then do speak to your psychiatrist or key worker about this. Many antipsychotic side effects can be controlled by diet and simple lifestyle changes or by other medications that can be prescribed for you. Alternatively, it may be possible to decrease the dose of the antipsychotic or to change over to a different antipsychotic. The principal side effects of four commonly prescribed atypical antipsychotics are summarized in Table 15.

Table 15:   Comparison of the side-effect profiles of four atypical antipsychotics

	Extrapyramidal side effects	Hyperpro-lactinaemia	Sedation	Weight gain	Orthostatic hypotension	Anticholinergic side effects
Risperidone	+	++	+	+	++	0/+
Olanzapine	0/+	+	++	+++	+	+/++
Quetiapine	0/+	0/+	++	++	++	0/+
Clozapine	0	0	+++	+++	+++	+++

Aripiprazole

Aripiprazole is a relatively recent, so-called third-generation antipsychotic that has been described as a 'dopamine-serotonin system stabiliser'. It is purported to have good efficacy in treating positive symptoms, negative symptoms, and mood symptoms, and to be better tolerated than other antipsychotics. Principal side effects include headache, anxiety, insomnia, nausea, vomiting, and light-headedness, but *not* extrapyramidal side effects, hyperprolactinaemia, sedation, or weight gain. As our understanding of schizophrenia improves, novel treatments such as aripiprazole are likely to continue emerging.

Antipsychotics in pregnancy and breastfeeding

There is some data to suggest that exposure to antipsychotic medication during the first trimester of pregnancy is linked to a small additional risk of congenital abnormalities in the foetus. At the same time, withholding antipsychotic medication may result in a relapse and in behavioural disturbances that expose the mother and foetus to much higher levels of overall risk. For this reason, pregnant women are generally advised to remain on their antipsychotic for the full duration of their pregnancy.

Antipsychotics are excreted into breast milk, but—except in the case of clozapine—breast-fed infants do not seem to suffer from this. Thus, a mother can decide to breast-feed whilst remaining on antipsychotic medication.

Taking antipsychotic medication

The starting dose of an antipsychotic is usually small so as to minimize any potential side effects. The dose is then increased according to the person's response, up to the smallest dose that is effective for that person. (This dose varies according to a large number of factors including age, sex, weight, and—of course—severity of symptoms).

What if the chosen antipsychotic is ineffective?

If a person does not respond to the chosen antipsychotic after a trial period of 6–8 weeks, the antipsychotic can be stopped and a different one started. If the person does not respond to two or more antipsychotics, an atypical antipsychotic called clozapine can be considered. Although clozapine is the most effective antipsychotic available, it requires registration with a monitoring service and, in the initial period, daily monitoring of vital signs (such as pulse rate and blood pressure) together with weekly blood tests. The purpose of the blood tests is to check the white blood cell count, which can drop dramatically in up to 1 per cent of people on clozapine. The role of white blood cells is to fight off infections, so a dramatic drop in the white blood cell count can leave the body exposed to all sorts of danger.

For how long should the antipsychotic be taken?

Antipsychotics not only combat the symptoms of schizophrenia, but also prevent them from re-occurring. If you have improved on a particular antipsychotic, you should continue taking it at the same dose for *at least* the next 6 months, preferably for the next 12–24 months, and possibly for much longer. Some schizophrenia sufferers remain on antipsychotic medication for several years and even several decades.

What if I have difficulties taking the antipsychotic?

Some people may be reluctant or unable to take their medication because, suffering from thought disorder or delusions, they do not realize or accept that they are ill. Other reasons for not taking medication include side effects, delusional beliefs about the medication (for example, that it is poison), fears of becoming addicted to the medication, poor concentration or motivation, and a poor relationship with the psychiatrist or key worker.

Missing tablets can precipitate a relapse or recurrence of symptoms, after which the schizophrenia sufferer may never quite regain the same level of functioning. After a first psychotic episode, three-quarters of people who stop taking their medication suffer from a relapse within 1 year, compared to less than half of those who continue to take their medication. For this reason, it is very important for both you and your family to discuss any difficulties in taking your medication and to have these difficulties addressed. For example, your psychiatrist may be able to reduce the dose of your antipsychotic, change your antipsychotic to a different one, or simplify your medication schedule.

Depot antipsychotics

Some people with persistent difficulties in taking their anti-psychotic medication may benefit from receiving it in the form of an injectable long-term preparation, or 'depot', instead of the usual oral tablet or oral liquid form. The principal advantages and disadvantages of depot versus oral antipsychotic medication are listed in Table 16. Before starting on a depot, it is usual to first be given an oral test dose. After about 7 days, the first depot dose is administered; the depot dose is then increased at regular intervals as the oral antipsychotic is decreased and stopped. Depot injections are usually administered every 7 or 14 days. The recently licensed paliperidone, which is the active metabolite of the older atypical antipsychotic risperidone, is administered once every 28 days.

The commonly used typical, atypical, and depot antipsychotics are listed in Table 17.

Table 16: Principal advantages and disadvantages of oral versus depot antipsychotics

	Advantages	*Disadvantages*
Oral medication	Short duration of action Flexible	Variable absorption from the gut Potential for poor compliance Potential for misuse and overdose
Depot medication	Less potential for poor compliance Less potential for abuse and overdose Regular contact with community psychiatric nurse or practice nurse, who gives the injection	Needle injections Potential delayed side effects Potential prolonged side effects Potential damage to relationship between the schizophrenia sufferer and his or her carers

Table 17:   Commonly used atypical, typical and depot antipsychotics

Antipsychotic	Trade name	Licensed daily dose range in adults under the age of 65 years
Atypical antipsychotics (introduced from 1990)		
Risperidone	Risperdal	2–16mg (rarely exceed 10mg)
Olanzapine	Zyprexa	5–20mg
Quetiapine	Seroquel	50–750mg (usual dose range 300–450mg)
Amisulpiride	Solian	400mg–1200mg
Clozapine	Clozaril/Denzapine	25–900mg (usual dose range 200–450mg)
Aripiprazole	Abilify	10–30mg
Typical antipsychotics (introduced from the 1950s)		
Chlorpromazine	Largactil	75–1000mg
Fluphenazine	Modecate/Moditen	2–20mg
Haloperidol	Haldol/Dozic/Serenace	3–30mg
Pimozide	Orap	2–20mg
Flupenthixol	Depixol	3–18mg
Zuclopenthixol	Clopixol	20–150mg
Sulpiride	Dolmatil/Sulpitil/Sulpor	400–2400mg
Depot antipsychotics		
Risperidone	Risperdal Consta	Maximum: 50mg every 2 weeks
Fluphenazine decanoate	Modecate	Test dose: 12.5mg; maximum: 100mg every 2 weeks
Flupenthixol decanoate	Depixol	Test dose: 20mg; maximum: 400mg/week
Zuclopenthixol decanoate	Clopixol	Test dose: 100mg; maximum: 600mg/week
Pipiotazine palmitate	Piportil depot	Test dose: 25mg; maximum: 200mg every 4 weeks

Augmentation

A minority of schizophrenia sufferers may not respond to a seemingly adequate trial of antipsychotic medication. This is often because of ongoing stressors in their life, because they are not taking the antipsychotic as prescribed, or because they are using substances such as cannabis or cocaine. If such factors have been excluded or addressed and the schizophrenia sufferer continues not to respond to his or her antipsychotic, another antipsychotic (often from a different class or group) should be tried. Sometimes, other medications such as a benzodiazepine, lithium, or carbamazepine may be prescribed alongside an antipsychotic to 'augment' its effect. Such augmentative strategies tend to be less effective than the antipsychotic clozapine, for which reason they are not usually recommended unless an adequate trial of clozapine has failed.

Keeping a treatment diary

It can be very helpful to keep a treatment diary in which you record the names and doses of the different medications that you have been on together with their major individual pros and cons. You and your psychiatrist can then use this treatment diary as a tool in choosing the best medication for you. See Table 18 for an example of such a treatment diary.

Table 18: My treatment diary

Medication	Dates taken	How taken	Positive effects	Side effects
Risperidone	15 January 2007 to 30 March 2007	Tablets Once a day before bed time	Voices almost disappeared Felt more relaxed Easy to take	Felt tired all day long Felt dizzy on standing up
Olanzapine	30 March 2007 to present	Tablets Once a day before bed time	Voices fully controlled Feel even more relaxed than on risperidone Easy to take	Initially put on 3kg (I have since lost this weight through diet and exercise)

8

Psychosocial treatments

The long-term care of a schizophrenia sufferer is usually planned at one or several multidisciplinary meetings which serve to establish the context of the illness, evaluate current personal circumstances, and formulate a detailed care plan to meet important medical, psychological, and social needs. As well as ensuring that the schizophrenia sufferer is receiving antipsychotic medication and is regularly reviewed by a member of the mental healthcare team, the care plan may in due course involve a number of psychosocial measures—possibly including patient and family education, family therapy, cognitive-behavioural therapy, illness self-management, self-help groups, and social and vocational skills training. Although under-utilized, these psychosocial measures together with a number of simple lifestyle changes can play an important role in containing symptoms, preventing relapse and re-hospitalization, and regaining a sense of control over your illness and, ultimately, your life goals and aspirations.

Expressed emotion

As you might recall from Chapter 2, 'expressed emotion' refers to critical, hostile, or emotionally overinvolved and overbearing attitudes directed at the schizophrenia sufferer by his or her relatives. These attitudes may take the form of critical comments and hostile or hurtful behaviours, and often originate in a misunderstanding that the schizophrenia sufferer is in control of his or her illness and simply 'choosing' to be ill. Alternatively, high expressed emotion might originate from an unjustified sense of guilt about the schizophrenia sufferer's illness or simply from a desire to be as helpful and proactive as possible. A number of studies have demonstrated that high expressed emotion from relatives and other carers is an important risk factor for schizophrenic relapse, even when it simply reflects legitimate distress and anxiety at the illness of a loved one.

Living in an environment with high expressed emotion is associated with as much as a fourfold increase in the rate of schizophrenic relapse. The pressure from close relatives in particular can be too much for the schizophrenia sufferer to bear, making him feel guilty, trapped, and helpless, and pushing him back into an acute psychosis. Expressed emotion is assessed by interviewing the schizophrenia sufferer and his close relatives, and, in some cases, by means of a taped family interview called the Camberwell Family Interview. Families with high expressed emotion may be offered educational sessions, stress management, or family therapy; each one of these interventions can help to reduce expressed emotion, and thereby form an important and integral part of the schizophrenia sufferer's care plan. Relatives who are educated about the nature of schizophrenia are better able to understand the needs and demands of their loved one, and therefore less likely to emit high expressed emotion. Although family therapy requires a considerable investment of time and effort, it may be especially appropriate if family members have fundamental difficulties in relating to one another.

Again, it cannot be stressed enough that families should not blame themselves for their loved one's illness. Instead, they should consider themselves as their loved one's greatest source of structure and support, and his or her greatest hope for a permanent recovery.

Cognitive-behavioural therapy

Developed by Aaron Beck in the 1960s, cognitive-behavioural therapy (CBT) is an increasingly common form of treatment for many psychiatric disorders. Although it is generally unsuitable in the management of acute psychosis, it can be helpful in the management of long-term, treatment-resistant symptoms and reduce the likelihood of relapse and re-hospitalization. It can also help to fight off depression and to enhance functional and social skills. CBT is most often carried out on a one-to-one basis but can also be offered in small groups. In either case, it involves a fixed number of sessions, typically about 10 to 20, each about an hour long. However, most of the 'work' takes place outside of sessions, and so requires a high degree of motivation on the part of the schizophrenia sufferer. The schizophrenia sufferer and a trained therapist (who may be either a psychologist, nurse, counselor, or doctor) develop a shared understanding of the schizophrenia sufferer's current problems and try to

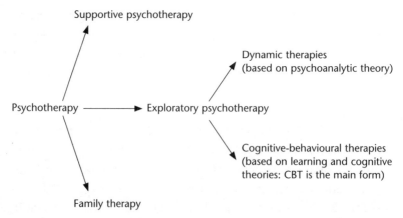

Figure 14:   Cognitive-behavioural therapy (CBT) in the context of psychotherapy as a whole. The three main forms of psychotherapy – supportive psychotherapy, exploratory psychotherapy (in the form of CBT), and family therapy – can all have a role to play in the management of schizophrenia. On balance, dynamic therapies based on psychoanalytic theory have not been proven effective in the management of schizophrenia.

explain them in terms of his or her thoughts, emotions, and behaviours. This leads to the identification of time-limited goals and of cognitive and behavioural strategies for achieving those goals. Thoughts are considered to be hypotheses that, through gentle questioning and guided discovery, can be examined, tested, and modified. Behavioural tasks might include self-monitoring, activity scheduling, graded assignments, and assertiveness training. In some cases, there may be an added focus on improving mood and self-esteem or on compliance with medication and relapse prevention.

Managing stress and anxiety

Stress and anxiety can make you much more vulnerable to a relapse in your illness. You might recall that stress can come from life events such as losing a loved one, going through a divorce, losing your job, or falling ill. But it can also come from seemingly smaller 'background' stressors such as constant deadlines, frustrations, and conflicts. The cumulative effect of such background stressors can be considerably greater than that of any single life event. The amount of stress that a person can comfortably handle is largely related to his or her coping and thinking styles and social skills. People with effective coping and thinking styles and good social skills are better able to diffuse stressful situations—for example, by doing something about them, putting them in their proper context, or simply talking about them and 'sharing the pain'.

The first step in dealing with stress is to be able to recognize its warning signs. Study Table 19 and then write down on a piece of paper how you feel when you become stressed. Next make a list of situations in which you feel that way. For each situation on your list, think about one or more strategies that you can use to make it less stressful.

Table 19:   Some of the symptoms of stress

Emotional symptoms	Anxiety, fear, irritability, anger, resentment, loss of confidence, depression
Psychological symptoms	Difficulty concentrating or making decisions, confusion, repetitive thoughts
Physical symptoms	Dry mouth, tremor, sweatiness, racing heartbeat, chest tightness and difficulty breathing, muscle tension, headache, dizziness
Behavioural symptoms	Nervous habits such as nail biting or pacing, drinking more coffee and alcohol, eating too much or too little, sleeping poorly, acting brashly or unreasonably, losing your temper, being inconsiderate of others, neglecting your responsibilities

Figure 15 lists stressful situations and a number of specific strategies for reducing the stress that relates to them. However, there are also more general strategies that can be used to reduce stress. One very effective strategy is deep breathing, which simply involves regulating your breathing: breathe in deeply

Stressful situations	Possible strategies for reducing stress
Arguing with Liz	Talk to Liz about how I am feeling and try to resolve matters
	See her less often
	Avoid talking to her about certain things
	Walk away from an argument
	Use deep breathing
Receiving bills that I can't pay	Ask a relative to help me with my finances
	Speak to a social worker to see what help I can get
	Phone the bank and try to reach an agreement

Figure 15:   Make a list of situations which you find stressful and for each situation think about one or more strategies for avoiding the situation or making it less stressful.

through your nose and hold in the air for several seconds. Then purse your lips and gradually let the air out, making sure that you let out as much air as you can. Keep on repeating this cycle until you are feeling more relaxed.

Another effective strategy, often used in conjunction with deep breathing, is physical relaxation. Lying flat on your back, tighten the muscles in your toes for 10 seconds and then relax them completely. Do the same for your feet, ankles, and calves, gradually moving up through your body until you reach your head and neck.

Other strategies that you can use for reducing stress include listening to classical music, taking a hot bath, reading a book or surfing the internet, calling up or meeting a friend, practicing yoga or meditation, and playing sports.

Lifestyle changes can help both to reduce stress and to increase your capacity to cope with stress. Lifestyle changes to consider include:

- Simplify your life, even if this means doing less or doing only one thing at a time
- Draw up a schedule and stick to it
- Get enough sleep
- Exercise regularly; for example, walking, swimming, yoga
- Eat a balanced diet
- Avoid excessive caffeine and alcohol
- Take time out to do the things that you enjoy doing
- Connect with others and share your problems with them
- Change your thinking style: have realistic expectations, reframe problems, express your feelings, maintain a sense of humour

These lifestyle changes are useful not only for managing stress, but also for improving your physical health and overall quality of life. Though individually small and simple, taken together and over time they can make a big difference to your chances of making a quick recovery and/or preventing a relapse.

If coping with stress continues to present a problem for you, consider asking a member of your mental healthcare team whether you can be sent for relaxation training.

Coping with voices

Sometimes voices can in themselves be a significant source of stress and distress. Simple strategies for reducing or eliminating voices include:

- Keep a diary of the voices to help you identify and avoid the situations in which they arise
- Find a trusted person with whom to discuss the voices
- Focus your attention on a distraction activity such as reading, gardening, singing, or listening to your favourite music
- Talk back at the voices: challenging them and asking them to go away. If out in public, you can avoid attracting attention to yourself by talking into a mobile phone
- Manage your anxiety and stress using the techniques discussed above
- Take your medication as prescribed, especially your anti-psychotic medication
- Avoid drugs and alcohol

Staving off depression

Depression affects as many as one in three schizophrenia sufferers. It can be difficult to distinguish the symptoms of depression from the negative symptoms of schizophrenia or the side effects of antipsychotic medication. The symptoms of depression are listed in Table 7 (see page 43). If you or your relatives suspect that you might be suffering from some of these symptoms, then do bring this to the attention of your mental healthcare team. It is important to have a high index of suspicion for depression and to seek advice sooner rather than later. Thanks to antidepressant medication and/or talking treatments, depression can be successfully treated.

Antidepressant medication

Antidepressants are commonly prescribed for the treatment of depression. Although they are not a solution to real life problems, they can improve your mood and make it easier to start dealing with real life problems. Modern antidepressants such as serotonin-selective reuptake inhibitors (SSRIs) improve mood by increasing the amount of the chemical messenger serotonin in the brain. Examples of SSRIs are citalopram, sertraline, fluoxetine, and paroxetine.

It is claimed that up to 70 per cent of people with depression respond to SSRIs. However, improvement in mood may be delayed for up to 10–20 days, so it is important not to give up on taking the tablets. Better sleep is often the first sign of improvement.

Like all medication, SSRIs can have side effects, but these are generally safer and more tolerable than those associated with older types of antidepressant. Common side effects of SSRIs include nausea, headache, dizziness, restlessness, and sedation. These side effects tend to be mild and to resolve within a few days or weeks. Some people may experience sexual dysfunction; as this side effect does not improve with time, it might require changing to another antidepressant.

After recovering from depression, it is important to keep on taking your SSRI at the same dose for at least another 6-9 months. People who have been on an SSRI for a long period of time and who abruptly stop taking it can suffer from flu-like symptoms. For this reason, SSRIs should be stopped gradually over a period of several days and weeks. If your SSRI fails to lift your mood, you can change to another SSRI or to a different type of antidepressant or ask to be referred for a psychological treatment.

Psychological treatments for depression

Although antidepressants are the most readily available form of treatment for depression, psychological or talking treatments can in many cases prove equally or even more effective. Schizophrenia sufferers often prefer talking treatments to antidepressants because they feel that the former address underlying problems rather than simply treat superficial symptoms. Types of talking treatment that are particularly suited for depression in schizophrenia are listed in Table 20. The type of talking treatment chosen depends on the schizophrenia sufferer's needs and preferences but also on the resources available in his or her local area. Opting for a talking treatment does not preclude being on an antidepressant, and there is some evidence to suggest that a talking treatment combined with an antidepressant can be more effective than either alone.

Table 20: Psychological or talking treatments that can be used for depression in schizophrenia

Psychological treatment	What it involves
Counselling	Identification and resolution of current life difficulties Explanation, resassurance, and support
Cognitive-behavioural therapy	Identification of thinking errors and associated behaviours that occur in depression Correction of these thinking errors and behaviours
Interpersonal psychotherapy	A systematic and standardized treatment approach to personal relationships and life problems that may be contributing to depression
Family therapy	Identification and resolution of negative aspects of family relationships that may be contributing to depression

Common thinking errors in depression

Some of the most important thinking errors (or 'cognitive distortions') in depression include,

- **Arbitrary inference**. Drawing a conclusion in the absence of evidence. An example is, 'The whole world hates me.'
- **Over-generalization**. Drawing a conclusion on the basis of limited and insufficient evidence. An example is, 'The shopkeeper gave me a cold glance. The whole world hates me.'
- **Magnification or minimization**. Over- or under-estimating the importance of an event. An example (of magnification) is, 'Now that my cat has died, I no longer have any reason to live.'
- **Selective abstraction**. Focussing on a single negative event or condition while ignoring other more positive ones. An example is, 'I'm not currently in a relationship (even though I have a loving family and many good friends).'
- **Dichotomous thinking**. 'All-or-nothing' thinking. An example is, 'If she doesn't come to see me today, then she doesn't love me (even tough she's thinking about me all the time but has no dependable means of transport).
- **Personalization**. Relating independent events to oneself. An example is, 'The nurse left her job because she was fed up looking after me.'
- **Catastrophic thinking**. Expecting disaster to strike at any minute. An example is, 'If I go out to the shops this afternoon I am more than likely to get run over.'

Things you can do to combat depression

There are a number of small and simple things that you can do to keep depression at bay.

- Ask your doctor for help, and try to stick with any medication that he or she prescribes
- Break large tasks into smaller ones, set yourself realistic goals for completing them, and don't take on more than you can manage

- Don't take any important decisions such as changing jobs or getting divorced while depressed. Thinking errors (see above) can easily lead you to make the wrong decision
- Spend time with other people and talk to them about how you are feeling. You can also phone a helpline such as SANEline for practical advice and support
- Let your family and friends help you. They may well be able to offer you the company, patience, affection, understanding, encouragement, and support that you need
- Get out of the house, even if only to buy a pint of milk or take a turn in the park
- Do more of the things that you usually enjoy doing: read a book, go to the shops or cinema, visit friends—anything that takes your mind off your negative thoughts is likely to make you feel better
- Take some mild exercise
- Get sufficient amounts of sleep. Even a single good night's sleep can leave you feeling much brighter
- Use the techniques discussed in a previous section to reduce stress and anxiety
- Challenge any negative thoughts—perhaps the most important thing of all. Make a list of all the positive things about yourself (you may need help with this), keep it on your person, and read it to yourself several times a day.

However bad you may be feeling, remember that you will not always be feeling this way. Have realistic expectations for yourself: improvements in mood are likely to be gradual rather than immediate, and there are going to be both good days and bad days.

Agree whom to call if you are overwhelmed by suicidal thoughts. This may be a relative or friend, a helpline, or your Community Mental Health Team. Carry the telephone numbers on you and make sure that you have one or several backups in case no one picks up your call.

Avoiding alcohol and drugs

Scientific research suggests that people who smoke cannabis are up to six times more likely to develop schizophrenia, and that people with schizophrenia who smoke cannabis have more frequent and more severe relapses of the illness. Other drugs that have been linked with schizophrenia include stimulant drugs such as amphetamines, ecstasy, and cocaine.

Having become ill, many schizophrenia sufferers turn to alcohol or illicit drugs such as cannabis, amphetamines, or cocaine to obtain relief from their symptoms and associated feelings of anxiety or depression. Alcohol and drugs may temporarily blunt or mask symptoms, but in the long term they are likely to lead to more frequent and severe relapses of the illness and to more profound anxiety and depression. You essentially create a 'vicious circle' in which the more you use alcohol and drugs to mask your symptoms, the worse your symptoms become; and the worse your symptoms become, the more you use alcohol and drugs to mask them. Using alcohol and drugs may also delay you from getting the help that you need, including getting a prescription for antipsychotic medication.

Consequences of alcohol or drug use

Possible consequences of using alcohol or drugs in schizophrenia sufferers include,

- Increased psychotic symptoms
- Reduced compliance with treatment
- Reduced response to treatment
- Increased risk of relapse and re-hospitalization
- Increased risk of depression and anxiety
- Medical complications such as high blood pressure, heart attack, stroke, stomach ulcers, and liver disease
- Complications of intravenous drug use such as hepatitis, HIV, infection, or venous thrombosis

- Familial and marital difficulties
- Employment difficulties
- Motoring offences
- Accidents
- Financial hardship
- Criminal activity and its consequences

Quitting alcohol and/or drugs

Simple advice and support is readily available from your Community Mental Health Team. For example, you can ask a healthcare professional to help you devise a goal-oriented management plan tailored to your needs. Tasks in this management plan could include, in the first instance, attending your appointments, keeping a diary of substance use, and taking your prescribed medication. Your relatives can play an important role in supporting and monitoring your progress and should, if possible, be included in the management plan. If relatives are included in the management plan, they should be advised to adopt an open and non-judgemental approach so as to bolster the self-esteem of their loved one and make him or her feel more in control of the problem.

Alcohol and drug use is frequently prompted by stressful situations, so learning techniques for managing stress and anxiety such as deep breathing and progressive muscle relaxation (see pages 75–78) can do much to decrease substance use. Also helpful is to rehearse and role play specific social skills that can then be deployed in stressful or high risk situations, for example, saying 'no' to a drug dealer or going into a pub and ordering a non-alcoholic drink.

If you find that you are in a stressful situation and about to give in, don't! Call a relative or carer, talk through the situation, and get the encouragement and support that you need to pull through. Some schizophrenia sufferers also find a great deal of encouragement and support in local support groups or in more structured 12-step programmes such as Alcoholics Anonymous or Narcotics Anonymous. Ask your psychiatrist or key worker if such groups may be suitable for you.

Alcoholics Anonymous

Founded in Ohio in 1935, Alcoholics Anonymous is a spiritually oriented community of alcoholics and reformed alcoholics with the common aims of staying sober and, through shared experience and understanding, helping others to do the same, 'one day at a time', by avoiding that first drink. The essence of the programme involves a 'spiritual awakening' achieved by 'working the steps', usually with the guidance of a more experienced member or 'sponsor'. Members initially attend daily meetings during which they share their experiences of alcoholism and recovery and engage in prayer and meditation. A prayer that is usually recited at every meeting is the Serenity Prayer, the short form of which goes,

> *God grant me the serenity to accept the things I cannot change,*
> *Courage to change the things I can,*
> *And the wisdom to know the difference.*

Taking care of your physical health

Being ill can promote a number of unhealthy habits and make it hard for you to change them. Taking care of your physical health not only increases your overall life expectancy and quality of life, but also promotes recovery and staves off negative feelings such as anxiety and depression. You create a virtuous circle whereby the better you feel, the better you are able to take care of your physical health; and the better you are able to take care of your physical health, the better you feel.

Compared with other groups of people, schizophrenia sufferers are more likely to eat poorly, lack exercise, and smoke heavily. They are therefore more likely to suffer from obesity;

diabetes; cardiovascular problems such as high blood pressure, heart attack, and stroke; and respiratory problems such as chronic bronchitis and emphysema. Some of the possible side effects of antipsychotic medication can directly or indirectly contribute to problems such as obesity and diabetes, making a healthy lifestyle that much more important.

Reasons for poor physical health in schizophrenia sufferers

Some of the common reasons for poor physical health in schizophrenia sufferers are,

- Poor diet
- Lack of exercise
- Smoking
- Alcohol and drug use
- Side effects of antipsychotic medication
- Social factors such as poor income and housing
- Poor monitoring of physical health

Of course, not all schizophrenia sufferers are plagued with poor physical health, but even so it is important that you have your physical health monitored on a regular basis so that any eventual problems can be picked up at an early stage and, hopefully, nipped in the bud. Your general practitioner is normally able to carry out a physical check at least once a year. This usually involves weighing you, taking your pulse rate and blood pressure, and carrying out a blood or urine test. A physical check is also a good opportunity to discuss your symptoms and medication and to obtain advice on issues such as diet, exercise, and smoking.

Eating the right diet

There are two separate factors to consider here,

- Whether you are eating the right amount (number of calories) to maintain your weight in the desirable range for health

- Whether you are eating the rights things to enjoy the benefits of a healthy, balanced diet

Consult the height-weight chart (Figure 16) to check whether you are the right weight for your height.

If you are underweight for your height, this may be a cause for concern and you should try to put on weight by eating sufficient quantities of a healthy, balanced diet. If this fails or if you have unintentionally lost a lot of weight, consult your general practitioner for further advice.

If you are overweight for your height, try to cut down on the amount you are eating, especially on foods that are high

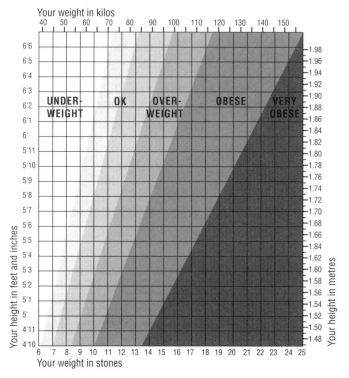

Figure 16: Height-weight chart.

in sugar and/or saturated and hydrogenated fats. Try also to take more exercise. If you are fat or very fat for your height, you are at a high risk of physical health problems such as diabetes, high blood pressure, heart problems, and stroke. It is especially important that you try to lose weight. At the same time, you need to be realistic about what can be achieved: rather than go on to a 'crash diet' that is bound to end in failure, aim to lose small amounts of weight steadily over a long period of time. Cut back on foods that are high in sugar or saturated and hydrogenated fats such as fizzy drinks, fried foods, meat products, hard cheese, cream, and butter. Eat three meals a day but avoid snacking in between meals, especially on 'comfort foods' such as chocolate, cakes, biscuits, and crisps. If you do feel like snacking, prefer a piece of fruit such as an apple, pear, or banana. If you have had problems with losing weight in the past, consult your general practitioner or a dietician for further advice.

If your weight is OK for your height, then you are most probably eating about the right amount to maintain your weight in the desirable range for health. This, however, does not necessarily mean that you are eating a healthy, balanced diet.

A healthy, balanced diet,

- Is based on starchy foods such as wholegrain bread, potatoes, pasta, and rice
- Contains a lot of fruit and vegetables (5 portions a day)
- Contains some protein-rich foods such as fish, poultry, meat, eggs, and pulses
- Is low in fat, sugar, and salt

Tips for eating well

Here are 8 tips for eating well from the UK Food Standards Agency consumer advice and information website (www.eatwell.gov.uk),

1. Base your meals on starchy foods
2. Eat lots of fruit and vegetables

3. Eat more fish
4. Cut down on saturated fat and sugar
5. Try to eat less salt—no more than 6g a day
6. Get active and try to be a healthy weight
7. Drink plenty of water
8. Don't skip breakfast

If you are eating a healthy, balanced diet, you are most probably getting all the vitamins and minerals that your body needs and do not need to take any dietary supplements.

Can schizophrenia be treated through diet?

Omega-3 fatty acids, found naturally in foods such as oily fish, linseed, and eggs, carry out a number of important functions in brain cells. A number of recent studies have suggested that omega-3 fatty acids may have benefits in schizophrenia if used as an adjunct to antipsychotic medication; however, larger scale research is required to confirm these findings. On the other hand, there is little evidence that schizophrenia can be treated through gluten-free or other special diets. If you intend to embark on a special diet or take dietary supplements, you should consult your general practitioner or psychiatrist for advice.

Getting enough exercise

Regular exercise is an important part of looking after both your physical and mental health. With regard to physical health, exercise helps you to lose weight and to maintain your target weight once you have reached it. It also decreases your blood pressure and increases your physical strength, endurance, and flexibility. Exercise usually improves the quality of your sleep, but should not be taken close to bedtime because of its short-term alerting effects.

With regard to mental health, exercise helps to decrease stress, improve thinking and motivation, boost self-esteem, and lift mood by causing the body to release increased amounts of chemical messengers called endorphins. Exercise also distracts you from positive symptoms such as hallucinations and delusions, and some studies of exercise in schizophrenia have reported beneficial effects on these symptoms.

Exercise does not have to be difficult or intensive; 30 minutes of moderate activity a day is all that you need to improve your fitness. You could do some gardening, walk to the shops, cycle, exercise at a gym or swimming pool, or play a team sport such as basketball or football. In fact, there are so many possibilities to choose from that you are bound to find one that you enjoy. By getting you out of the house and 'out of yourself', exercise can remove you from emotional conflict, distract you from your symptoms, and increase the number and frequency of your social interactions. This in itself can have an important salutary effect on your mental health.

The various benefits of exercise in people with schizophrenia are summarized in Table 21.

Table 21:   Some of the benefits of exercise in schizophrenia

Weight loss
Improved physical strength, endurance and flexibility
Decreased stress
Decreased blood pressure
Better sleep
Improved thinking
Improved motivation
Better mood
Better self-esteem
Distraction from positive symptoms
Removal from emotional conflict
Increased social interactions

Getting enough sleep

Insomnia—difficulty in falling asleep or remaining asleep for long enough—affects about 30 per cent of the general population and an even greater proportion of schizophrenia sufferers, in whom it can present as a direct effect of the illness. Insomnia can also be caused or aggravated by poor sleeping habits, depression, anxiety, stress, physical problems such as pain or breathing difficulties, medication, and substance use (Table 22). Short-term insomnia in particular is often caused by a stressful life event, a poor sleep environment, or an irregular routine. Insomnia is usually a problem if it occurs on most nights and causes distress or daytime effects such as fatigue, poor concentration, poor memory, and irritability. These symptoms may postpone your recovery and also predispose you to accidents, psychiatric complications such as anxiety and depression, and medical problems such as high blood pressure, infections, obesity, and diabetes.

Table 22:   Some of the commoner causes of insomnia

Poor sleep habits
Psychiatric disorders
       Depressive disorder
       Mania and bipolar affective disorder
       Anxiety disorders
       Schizophrenia
       Post-traumatic stress disorder
       Chronic fatigue syndrome
Medical disorders
       Restless leg syndrome (thrashing about during sleep)
       Sleep apnoea (snoring with pauses in breathing during sleep)
       Chronic pain
       Chronic obstructive pulmonary disease
       Chronic renal failure
       Neurological disorders such as Parkinson's disease and other movement
          disorders
       Headaches
       Fibromyalgia
Other
       Alcohol and drug misuse
       Side effects of medication such as antipsychotic or antidepressant
          medication
       Shift working
       Caring for young children

If you are suffering from insomnia, there are a number of simple measures that you can take to resolve or at least reduce the problem.

- Enforce a strict routine involving regular and adequate sleeping times (most adults need about 7–8 hours sleep every night). Allocate a time for sleeping, for example, 11pm to 7am, and do not use this time for any other activities. Avoid daytime naps, or make them short and regular. If you have a bad night, avoid 'sleeping in' as this will only make it more difficult to fall asleep the following night.
- Implement a bedtime routine that enables you to relax and 'wind down' before going to bed. This may involve doing breathing exercises or meditation or simply reading a book, listening to music, or watching TV. Many people find it helpful to have a hot drink: if this is the case for you, prefer a herbal or malted or chocolaty drink to stimulant drinks such as tea or coffee.
- Sleep in a familiar, dark, and quiet room that is adequately ventilated and neither too hot nor too cold. Try to use this room for sleeping only so that your mind comes to associate it with sleep.
- If you can't sleep, don't become anxious and try to force yourself to fall asleep. The more anxious you become, the less likely you are to fall asleep, and this is only likely to make you more anxious! Instead, get up and do something relaxing and enjoyable for about half an hour and then try again.
- Take regular exercise during the daytime, but do not exercise in the evening or close to bedtime because the short-term alerting effects of exercise may make it more difficult to fall asleep.
- Try to reduce your overall levels of stress by implementing some of the simple lifestyle changes detailed on page 77.
- Eat an adequate evening meal containing a good balance of complex carbohydrates and proteins. Eating too much can

make it difficult to fall asleep; eating too little can disturb your sleep and decrease its quality.

- Avoid caffeine, alcohol, and tobacco, especially in the evening. Also avoid stimulant drugs such as cocaine, amphetamines, and ecstasy. Alcohol may make you fall asleep more easily, but it also decreases the quality and duration of your sleep.

If insomnia persists despite these measures, seek advice from your general practitioner or psychiatrist. In some cases, insomnia may have a clear and definite cause that needs to be addressed—for example, a physical problem or a side effect of medication (see Table 22). Behavioural interventions such as sleep restriction therapy or cognitive-behavioural therapy can be helpful in some cases and are generally preferable to sleeping tablets. Although they may be effective in the short term, sleeping tablets are problematic in the longer term because they become impossible to do without (an effect called dependence) and because ever-higher doses are required to produce the same benefit (an effect called tolerance). Sleeping remedies that are available without a prescription often contain an antihistamine that can leave you feeling drowsy the following morning. If you decide to use such remedies, it is important that you do not drive or operate heavy machinery the next day. Herbal alternatives are usually based on valerian, a hardy perennial flowering plant with heads of sweetly scented pink or white flowers. If you are thinking about using a herbal remedy, do speak to your general practitioner or psychiatrist first, particularly if you have a medical condition or allergy, are already on medication, or are pregnant or breastfeeding.

Quitting cigarettes

Schizophrenia sufferers are nearly three times as likely to smoke as the average person, a higher incidence than in any other mental illness. They are also more likely to smoke heavily, with dire consequences for their physical health, quality of life, and life expectancy. Indeed, the most common causes of death in people with schizophrenia are not the direct effects of the illness but cardiovascular and respiratory diseases that are caused or aggravated by smoking. Smoking also causes a drop in blood levels of antipsychotic medication, such that smokers require higher doses of antipsychotic medication than non-smokers to benefit from the same therapeutic effect. Assuming that a pack of 20 cigarettes costs an average of £7.46, someone on 40 cigarettes a day spends about £5445.80 on cigarettes every year. Although roll-up cigarettes are cheaper than filter cigarettes, they can be even more damaging to your physical health.

Most schizophrenia sufferers who smoke started doing so before their illness began, suggesting either that smoking pre-disposes to schizophrenia or, more plausibly, that the genetic and environmental factors that predispose to schizophrenia also predispose to nicotine addiction. An alternative and more convincing explanation for the high incidence of smoking in schizophrenia sufferers is that their illness or disposition makes them more likely to smoke, either because smoking helps them to relax or because it alleviates symptoms such as hallucinations and confusion.

A commonly held perception is that schizophrenia sufferers are unlikely to give up smoking and that it is unreasonable or even unfair to try to deprive them of one of their principal pleasures and pastimes. The truth is that many schizophrenia sufferers are highly motivated to stop smoking and in need of all the help they can get to fight off what is often a severe nicotine addiction. Help can take the form of smoking cessation groups, behavioural therapy, nicotine replacement (for example, in the form of patches or lozenges), and alternative therapies such as acupuncture and hypnosis. Success rates vary from one person to the next, but it is important to keep on persisting.

If you are motivated to stop smoking, mention this to your general practitioner or psychiatrist. You can also find further information and support at www.netdoctor.co.uk/smoking/index.shtml.

How to stop smoking

Make a list of the pros and cons of smoking. See Table 23 for an example of such a list. Keep your list on your person and read it several times a day to motivate yourself to quit. Choose a date on which you want to quit and stick to it. Between now

Table 23:   Pros and cons of smoking

Pros	Cons
Makes it easier to socialize with other smokers	Constant nagging from my partner
	Bad breath putting my partner off
Makes me feel more confident in social situations	Constantly having to go outside, even in the cold and rain
Provides me with momentary gratification	The rancid smell in my house and on my clothes
Prevents cravings and withdrawal symptoms	The effects on my health: sore throat, cough, shortness of breath, high blood pressure, stomach ulcers
	The effects on my appearance: looking 10 years older than I really am with yellow teeth, fingernails and skin
	Intense craving and withdrawal symptoms if I don't smoke
	Always needing a fix, and being unable to simply relax and enjoy life
	Feelings of inadequacy for not giving up
	Feelings of fear and anxiety at what I am doing to myself and how it will all end
	Feelings of guilt for the passive smoking endured by those around me
	The cost of it all, especially the fact that I can never afford a holiday

and that date, keep a log of your smoking habits: record the times at which you 'light up', where you then were, what you were doing, and how you were feeling. Use this log to gain a better understanding of your smoking habits. Once your chosen date arrives, make a clean break by throwing out all cigarettes and removing all ashtrays, lighters, and matches. You are then likely to experience intense cravings together with withdrawal symptoms such as irritability, difficulty concentrating, tiredness, headache, increased appetite, and insomnia. Nicotine replacement can help to relieve these cravings and withdrawal symptoms, so do ask your general practitioner or psychiatrist to prescribe some for you. Cravings rarely last for more than a couple of minutes at a time and diversion techniques such as chewing gum, brushing your teeth, or playing a video game may take your mind off them until they pass. If these diversion techniques fail, call a friend or relative who knows what you are going through and is willing to give you some support. Alternatively, take another look at your list of pros and cons and use it to keep yourself motivated. Cravings are often triggered by certain places, activities, and emotions that you have come to associate with smoking. Use the log of your smoking habits to identify these places, activities, and emotions, and try to devise alternative coping strategies.

Remember that cravings and withdrawal symptoms do not last forever, and that in a matter of only days quitting will have become a much easier task! Do not be too harsh on yourself if you give in to temptation: put it behind you and keep on trying your best.

Coping with stigma

One of the most difficult challenges for those recovering from schizophrenia is coping with the reactions of other people. Mental illness in general and schizophrenia in particular attract a great deal of stigma from the general public. This is in large part due to ignorance and the fear that is born out of it, a fear that is reinforced by the misrepresentation of schizophrenia sufferers in the media. Once again, schizophrenia sufferers do not have split personalities, and as a group are neither unpredictable nor dangerous. They are not lazy or 'moral failures', and getting better is not simply a matter of them 'pulling themselves together'. Mental illnesses, like all medical conditions, have a biological basis and are not simply 'all in the mind'.

Some highly creative people have suffered from schizophrenia, including Syd Barrett, the early driving force behind the rock band Pink Floyd; John Nash, the father of 'game theory'; and Vaslav Nijinsky, the legendary choreographer and dancer. Similarly, many highly creative people have had close relatives with schizophrenia including the physicist Albert Einstein (his son), the philosopher Bertrand Russell (also his son), and the novelist James Joyce (his daughter). It has even been suggested that the genes that predispose to schizophrenia also confer an important adaptive advantage to mankind, namely, the abilities for language and creativity—an idea that I discuss at much greater length in my book, *The Meaning of Madness*.

Stigma can create a vicious cycle of alienation and discrimination that hinders progress to recovery by promoting social isolation, stress, depression, alcohol and drug misuse, unemployment, homelessness, and institutionalization. Sadly, many schizophrenia sufferers report that stigma is just as distressing as the actual symptoms of their illness. In some cases, they fear stigma so much that they refuse to accept that they are ill and as a result do not seek out the help that they so desperately need.

For these reasons, it is especially important that carers analyse their attitudes and behaviours and make doubly sure that they are not involuntarily contributing to the stigmatization of the person whom they are caring for. Attitudes and behaviours that contribute to stigma are often subtle, and may, for example, involve talking to the schizophrenia sufferer louder than necessary, talking about him as though he were not in the room, and failing to grant him sufficient independence and responsibility. A simple rule of thumb for carers is to behave towards the schizophrenia sufferer as they would to any other person: naturally, simply, and with due respect and courtesy. Carers should try to become a 'refuge' or 'comfort zone' for the person whom they are caring for, offering him or her practical and emotional support but also the space and time to be quiet and alone. Deep questioning, argument, and the venting of intense negative emotions are only likely to overwhelm the schizophrenia sufferer.

Many schizophrenia sufferers feel unable to talk about their illness for fear of the pain and shame of being stigmatized. Being open about your illness might be a risk, but it also enables you to talk through your feelings and get the support that you need. Learn as much as you can about the illness so that you can correct any false beliefs that people may hold about it. Try to educate friends and relatives about the illness and the issues surrounding it. If people use derogatory terms such as 'schizo' or 'psycho', remind them that their behaviour is unacceptable. If you feel that you are being unfairly treated as a customer or service user, get empowered and make a complaint. You can even take a public stance against discrimination, for example, by speaking at events or writing about your experiences on a blog or even in a bulletin, magazine, or newspaper. Joining a local support group enables you to meet other schizophrenia sufferers and, at least temporarily, to escape from stigma.

Preventing relapses

A relapse in illness can have devastating consequences for the schizophrenia sufferer and his or her loved ones. After each relapse, it becomes increasingly difficult to regain control over your symptoms, and each relapse also has important repercussions on your long-term outcome and quality of life. For these reasons, you must do everything in your power to prevent a relapse.

There is strong scientific evidence that long-term treatment with antipsychotic medication substantially reduces rates of relapse and re-hospitalization in schizophrenia. If you are reluctant to take your antipsychotic because the schedule is too complicated or because you are suffering from troublesome side effects, then do speak to your psychiatrist about this. He or she may be able to simplify the schedule, decrease the dose, or change you over to an antipsychotic that suits you better. Do not simply stop taking your medication in the hope that everything will be fine. If, after several years, you do decide to come off your medication, this should be done gradually and cautiously with plenty of support and monitoring from your mental healthcare team. Taking your medication at the dose prescribed by your psychiatrist is the single most important thing that you can do to prevent a relapse in your illness—unfortunate, but there it is.

People with schizophrenia and their carers need to learn to recognize the early signs and symptoms of a relapse. These signs and symptoms may differ from person to person, but common ones include:

- Suffering changes in mood
- Losing your sense of humour
- Becoming tense, irritable, or agitated
- Finding it difficult to concentrate
- Retreating from social situations and neglecting outside activities and social relationships
- Becoming increasingly suspicious or hostile
- Saying or doing irrational, inappropriate, or otherwise unusual things
- Developing strange or fantastical ideas
- Neglecting your personal care

- Omitting to take your medication
- Dressing in inappropriate or unusual clothes or combinations of clothes, for example, wearing sunglasses indoors
- Sleeping excessively or hardly at all, and/or at unusual times of the day
- Eating excessively or hardly at all
- Becoming especially sensitive to noise or light
- Hearing voices or seeing things that other people cannot hear or see

If any of these signs and symptoms should rear their heads, contact your local mental healthcare team immediately for support and advice—this might just help you to avert a full-scale relapse. It is a good idea to have an action plan in place before problems arise and to have discussed this plan with your local mental healthcare team. You can also keep a diary of your thoughts, feelings, and doings to help you and your carers identify the signs and symptoms of a relapse. In the event of a relapse, your thinking may become severely impaired and you may have to simply trust in the judgement of your carers.

Finally, try to identify any factors that may have caused or contributed to your difficulties, since addressing these factors may also help in averting a full-scale relapse. Some of the most important relapse factors are listed in Table 24 and discussed more fully in other sections of this book. Keeping them under control can help you to prevent a relapse and so to improve your chances of a complete and permanent recovery.

Table 24:   Some of the most important factors that may cause or contribute to a schizophrenic relapse

Non-compliance with medication or decreased dose of medication (see pages 67–68)

Alcohol and drugs (see pages 84–85)

High expressed emotion (see pages 72–73)

Stress (see pages 75–78)
Depression and anxiety (see pages 78–82)
Stigma (see pages 96–98)
Lack of social relationships and support
Poor physical health (see pages 85–90)
Lack of sleep (see pages 90–93)
Poor understanding of schizophrenia in general, and of signs of symptoms of relapse in particular

Caring, and caring for carers

Each year in the UK over two million people take up a caring role, so as a carer you are certainly not alone. A good carer can be a schizophrenia sufferer's most invaluable source of structure and support and his or her greatest hope for a permanent recovery. Though you may feel that caring for a loved one is more a duty than a job, you should identify yourself as a carer so that you can obtain the help and support that you are entitled to. Try to learn as much as you can about schizophrenia and to have a good idea of how it might affect your loved one. For example, your loved one may not be spontaneous in his responses to your questions. This is not because he is ignoring you, but because his thoughts are confused and/or he is being distracted by voices. Understanding the illness builds up your confidence as a carer and gives you a clearer sense of what you might and might not be able to achieve. Remember that there is only so much you alone can do to help your loved one: being realistic about your aims helps to avert guilt, prevent conflict, manage stress, and avoid burn-out. Ask your local mental healthcare team for further information about schizophrenia and, in particular, for specific advice about caring for your loved one. Information and advice is also available from voluntary organizations such as the ones listed under 'Useful addresses'—and, of course, there is plenty of it in this book.

Caring for your loved one is likely to require a lot of patience: schizophrenia sufferers have good days and bad days and tend to make progress in small steps. A relapse in the illness is likely to sap your morale and it is important that you be prepared for this. It is a good idea to have an action plan in place before problems arise and to have discussed this plan both with your loved one and with the local mental healthcare team. If problems do arise, contact the mental healthcare team sooner rather than later, as it may still be possible to contain the situation and avoid a full-scale relapse. Remember that your caring role has made you an important source of information and expertise: learn to rely on your previous experiences and to trust in your instinct or judgement. At the same time, try to involve your loved one in making decisions about his or her care.

Sometimes a schizophrenia sufferer may fail to recognize that he or she is ill, and so refuse to engage with carers or the mental healthcare team. In particular, he or she may insist that delusions and hallucinations are real or feel too paranoid to trust in anyone. If your loved one is refusing to engage with the mental healthcare team, you can try to break the prospect of treatment into smaller, more manageable steps, starting with an initial appointment. If possible, give your charge a degree of choice in booking the appointment and propose that you or someone else comes along.

As progress is usually made in small steps, it is all too easy for carers to lose sight of the fact that progress is actually being made. Try to feel positive about your loved one and to gently encourage and facilitate his or her progress. One of the most important things that you can do as a carer is to ensure that your loved one takes his or her antipsychotic medication as prescribed. Be on the lookout for any potential side effects (see pages 62–66), and do not hesitate to report these to your local mental healthcare team. Another important thing that a carer can do is to try to establish a simple daily structure and routine with regular eating and sleeping times. Last but not least, do encourage your charge to attend appointments with the mental healthcare team and other services.

But, avoid nagging, criticizing, telling off, shouting, arguing, and other manifestations of expressed emotion. Do not lose sight of the fact that high expressed emotion is an important predictor of relapse in schizophrenia and ensure that you are giving your loved one sufficient time and space to get better. This can be difficult to achieve, as it is often a carer's instinct to do as much as possible for their loved one and many carers have unrealistic expectations about the progress that he or she ought to be making. If you feel that this is a particular issue for you as a carer, then do speak to your mental healthcare team about it. Families with high expressed emotion can be offered educational sessions, stress management, or family therapy, all of which can help to deflate expressed emotion and form an important and integral part of the care plan.

Finally, do not neglect other family members. Brothers and sisters of schizophrenia sufferers, particularly if they are young, may feel that they are no longer getting their fair share of parental attention and may become envious and resentful.

Looking after your health

Carers need to care for themselves if they are to care most effectively for another. Many carers come under severe stress and suffer from serious health problems such as heart disease or mental illness. It is important that you recognize this and take it seriously if you are not to become ill and unable to fulfil your role as a carer. Use some of the techniques for stress management listed on pages 75–78 to reduce your levels of stress and arrange for an annual health check-up with your general practitioner. Make sure that you look after yourself, that you plan and pursue activities that you enjoy, and that you take a break or holiday from caring if you feel that you need one.

Getting the support that you need

Remember that you are not alone as a carer: share your opinions and experiences with the mental healthcare team looking after your loved one and feel free to ask individual team members for help and advice. Conversely, your perspective on your loved one is invaluable to the team, so try to attend and participate in any meetings or consultations about his or her care. Identify someone that you can talk to on a more personal level (perhaps a close friend or relative) about your experiences as a carer. Some friends and relatives may find it difficult to discuss your caring role and may underestimate the efforts that you are making as a carer. The onus is on you to broach the subject and enlist their help and support. Joining a local carers' support group enables you to feel that you are not alone in your carer role and provides you with an invaluable opportunity to learn from the good and bad experiences of others carers. It can also help you to understand any negative emotions that you may be harbouring— for example, guilt, shame, anger, or helplessness—and to prevent these emotions from interfering with the care of your loved one.

Avoiding blame

Some carers think that schizophrenia is caused by poor parenting, and fear they are to blame for their son or daughter's illness. Their feelings of guilt can come to dominate family life and add to the heavy burden already carried by their child. In the 1940s some psychoanalysts believed that certain mental illnesses such as schizophrenia and autism resulted from being born to a 'refrigerator mother', that is, an emotionally absent and therefore inadequate mother. This theory and other similar theories have never found scientific backing and have long since been discredited and discarded. In fact, scientific research increasingly indicates that schizophrenia is, in the main, a biological illness of the brain.

Some carers may look around for someone else to blame for their son or daughter's illness, such as the general practitioner, the psychiatrist, or even their very son or daughter. That they should do so is natural and understandable, since it helps them to make sense of the terrible illness of a loved one. Nonetheless, they should remember that the real 'culprit' is ultimately a biological illness of the brain. Instead of playing the blame game, they should focus their energies on the road to recovery.

Dealing with anger

Like guilt and blame, frustration and anger can be a normal reaction to the illness of a loved one. Parents often have thoughts such as, 'Why did this happen to our family?' or even, 'Why should I bother any more? I can't put up with all the hard work and, ultimately, it's all going to be for nothing.' Sometimes parents may direct their anger and frustration at their child even though they realize that he or she is not to blame for the illness. Unchecked anger adds to your stress and to that of your child and thereby prevents your family from getting ahead. Although you cannot change the reality of the illness, you can change your attitude and reaction to it. Try diffusing your anger by talking about the feelings that underlie it: talk to friends, relatives, mental healthcare professionals, and other families afflicted by schizophrenia. Or else try channelling your anger so that it becomes a force for good, for example, motivating you to read up about the illness or to seek help for your family.

Getting extra help

You can obtain an assessment of your needs as a carer simply by asking your general practitioner to refer you to local Social Services or by directly referring yourself. A carer's needs assessment can be instrumental in ensuring that your practical needs as a carer are met. You can find out more about the carer support services available in your area through Social Services, through a local carers' organization, or through Carers UK and their dedicated phone line, CarersLine. Such services may include help at home, aids and equipment, break services, and day care, among others.

Many carers are reluctant to claim social benefits, either because they have never done so before or because they are put off by complicated rules and difficult forms. As a carer you play an important role in society and the benefits that you are entitled to exist to recognize and support that role. These benefits are detailed on pages 108–110. You can get help in claiming them from your local mental healthcare team, local Social Services, or voluntary organizations such as Carers UK.

Carrying on with life outside of your caring role

Being a carer can be so stressful and demanding that it just takes over your life. It is crucial that you also think about yourself and about your future, particularly since a time may come when you are no longer required to be a carer. As the condition of your loved one improves, he or she may become more independent and, in some cases, move out to an apartment or group home. When this happens, carers often find themselves lacking in purpose and direction and unable to adjust to their sudden change of circumstances. For this and other reasons, it is important that you continue to plan and pursue activities that you enjoy and, essentially, keep up your life outside of your caring role. Many carers find the time to commit to a part-time job, which can represent both a salutary distraction from the burdens of caring and an invaluable source of additional income. Others take the opportunity to further their skills, for example, by enrolling for evening classes or even a part-time degree.

Caring for siblings

As parents focus their attention on their ill son or daughter, they naturally run the risk of being less available to their other children. However, these other children are likely to be profoundly affected by the illness of their sibling and more in need of parental attention than ever. In particular, they may be fearful for their family and/or anxious of developing the illness themselves. Schizophrenia often strikes in the prime of life, at a time when young people are launching into life—starting college or university, getting a first job, or enjoying and expanding their range of activities and relationships. Siblings may find it difficult to savour their successes while witnessing their ill brother or sister slipping further and further behind. At the same time, they may feel pressured to achieve more so as to 'compensate' for their brother or sister's illness and not add to the burden of their afflicted parents.

Siblings should not blame themselves or anybody else for their brother or sister's illness or let it prevent them from partaking in life outside of the family. By nurturing old friendships, they should be able to obtain support and talk through difficult feelings such as anger, anxiety, and guilt. Tough though the situation may be, parents need to make a special effort to cater to the needs of siblings and to ensure as far as possible that they are included in family discussions surrounding the illness. Conversely, if siblings feel that they are not getting the parental attention that they need, they should not feel afraid to raise this as an issue. Siblings should educate themselves as much as possible about the illness, and, depending on their age, also consider joining a carers' support group. Older siblings may play an active role in caring and, in so doing, provide their parents with much needed respite.

Driving and schizophrenia

You should stop driving during a first psychotic episode or psychotic relapse of your illness so as not to endanger your life and the lives of others. In the UK, you must notify the Driver and Vehicle Licensing Agency (DVLA): failure to do so makes it illegal for you to drive and invalidates your insurance. The DVLA will then send you a medical questionnaire to fill out together with a form asking for your permission to contact your psychiatrist. Your driving licence can generally be reinstated if your psychiatrist can confirm that,

- Your illness has been successfully treated with medication for a period of at least 3 months
- You are conscientious about taking your medication
- Any side effects that you are suffering from are not likely to impair your driving
- You are not using illegal drugs

Further information on schizophrenia and driving can be found on the DVLA website, www.dvla.gov.uk. Note that the rules for professional driving are different from—and more stringent than—those detailed above.

Social benefits

Every year in the UK, millions of pounds of social benefits are left unclaimed, often by people with a mental illness and their carers. The state benefits available to you are detailed here. For further information on these, see the Department for Work and Pensions website, www.dwp.gov.uk/lifeevent/benefits, contact your local Citizens Advice Bureau, or get in touch with local Social Services.

Housing Benefit and Council Tax Benefit

Housing Benefit and Council Tax Benefit are means-tested, tax-free payments made to people who need help with paying the rent and council tax on their property. From 1st January 2012, if you are single and under 35, you can only get housing benefit for bed-sit accommodation or one room in shared accommodation. Both Housing Benefit and Council Tax Benefit are administered by the local authority of the area in which your property, bedsit, or room is located. Note that these benefits cannot cover mortgage interest payments.

Income Support

Income Support is a means-tested payment made to people between the ages of 16 and 59 who work less than 16 hours a week and who have a reason for not actively seeking work (on grounds of disability, caring for children, or caring for relatives). Claimants of Income Support are also entitled to other benefits such as Housing Benefit and Council Tax Benefit (see above).

Social fund

Social fund payments are payments, grants, or loans made in addition to certain benefits for intermittent expenses that cannot be met by normal income.

Employment and Support Allowance

From 31 January 2011, people under State pension age with an illness or disability that restricts their ability to work are required to apply for Employment and Support Allowance rather than Incapacity Benefit. Employment and Support Allowance involves not only financial help but also, if appropriate, support to get back into some kind of employment.

Disabled person's tax credit

The disabled person's tax credit is for people beyond the age of 16 who work an average of 16 hours a week or more and who have an illness or disability that restricts the amount that they can earn.

Disability Living Allowance

Disability Living Allowance is paid to people under the age of 65 who are in need of personal care or help with getting around or both. It is not means-tested. Note that from 2013, people of working age (16–64) will need to apply for the new Personal Independence Payment, which will be based on the impact rather than the nature of the disability.

Attendance Allowance

Attendance Allowance is paid to people aged 65 or more who need help with personal care because of an illness or disability. It is not means-tested.

NHS costs

Depending on your circumstances, you may qualify for free NHS prescriptions and hospital medicines, free NHS dental treatment, and free NHS eyesight tests. Other NHS costs may also be met.

Carer's Allowance

Carer's Allowance is a means-tested, taxable weekly benefit payment for people who care for someone in receipt of Attendance Allowance or Disability Living Allowance at the middle or high rate of care. Among other stipulations, the carer must be over 16 years of age and spend 35 hours a week or more in his or her caring role. The carer does not have to be related to or living with the person for whom he or she is caring.

Useful addresses

Carers UK

20 Great Dover Street
London SE 1 4LX
Carers Line: 0808 808 7777 (FOC, 10–12am & 2–4pm, Weds, Thurs)
Website: www.carersuk.org

Carers give so much to society. Yet, as a consequence of caring, they can experience ill health, poverty, and discrimination. Carers UK seeks to end this injustice by mobilizing carers and supporters, campaigning for change, carrying out research, and transforming the public perception of what caring is about.

Crisis

66 Commercial Street
London E1 6LT
Tel. 0300 636 1967
Website: www.crisis.org.uk

Crisis provides help and support to homeless people or people in danger of becoming homeless so that they can escape the cycle of homelessness and rebuild their lives.

Depression Alliance

20 Great Dover Street
London SE1 4LX
Tel. 0845 123 2320
Website: www.depressionalliance.org

The leading UK charity for people with depression, Depression Alliance provides services including publications, supporter services, local self-help groups, and a pen-friend scheme. It also carries out research into depression, raises public awareness of the condition, and campaigns for changes to mental health policy and practices.

Making Space

Lyne House
46 Allen Street
Warrington
Cheshire WA2 7JB
Tel. 01925 571 680
Website: www.makingspace.co.uk

Making Space provides support to people with a physical or mental illness, learning difficulties, or dementia. It also provides support to their carers. Services offered include family intervention services, rehabilitative employment and education services, supported housing, care homes, residential accommodation, clinical services, computerised cognitive behavioural therapy, and extra care services.

Mind (National Association for Mental Health)

15–19 Broadway
London E15 4BQ
Mind infoline: 0300 123 3393 (local call, 9am–6pm, Mon–Fri)
Website: www.mind.org.uk

Mind offers information and advice to people with mental health problems and lobbies government and local authorities on their behalf. It also works to raise public awareness and understanding of issues relating to mental health. Over 160 local Mind associations (independent, affiliated charities) provide services such as supported housing, floating support schemes, care homes, drop-in centres, and self-help support groups. The information line offers confidential help and a special legal service.

Rethink (formerly the National Schizophrenia Fellowship)

89 Albert Embankment
London SE1 7TP
Advice team: info@rethink.org or 0300 5000 927 (local call,
    10am–1pm, Mon–Fri)
Website: www.rethink.org

Rethink Mental Illness helps almost 60,000 people every year. Its offers services across a large number of areas, including advocacy, carer support, community support, criminal justice, crisis, employment and training, helpline and advice, housing, nursing and residential care, and talking treatments.

The Royal College of Psychiatrists

Website: www.rcpsych.ac.uk.mentalhealthinformation.aspx

The Royal College of Psychiatrists is a professional and educational organization for psychiatrists in the UK and Republic of Ireland. It produces a range of high-quality materials for the general public, including various leaflets on schizophrenia and treatments such as CBT and depot antipsychotic medication. The link above should lead you directly to the mental health information portal.

Samaritans

The Upper Mill
Kingston Road
Ewell
Surrey KT17 2AF
Helpline: 08457 90 90 90 (1.021p/min off-peak, 24/7)
Website: www.samaritans.org

Samaritans provides confidential, non-judgemental support to anyone in emotional distress or at risk of suicide. At its core is a telephone helpline, operating 24 hours a day, 365 days a year.

In addition, it offers a drop-in service for face-to-face discussion, undertakes outreach at festivals and other outdoor events, trains prisoners as 'Listeners', and carries out research into suicide and emotional health issues.

SANE (Schizophrenia A National Emergency)

First Floor
Cityside House
40 Adler Street
London E1 1EE
Helpline: 0845 676 8000 (local call, 6–11pm, 7/7)

SANE combats stigma, campaigns to improve mental healthcare services, and provides emotional support to people with mental health problems and their carers. It also initiates research into the causes and treatments of serious mental illness. The SANE helpline provides information, emotional support, and crisis care to people with mental health problems and their carers. Calls may be anonymous.

The Sleep Council

High Corn Mill
Chapel Hill
Skipton
North Yorkshire BD23 1NL
Freephone leaflet line: 0800 018 2923
Website: www.sleepcouncil.com

The Sleep Council provides useful general advice on sleep and beds.

Alcoholics Anonymous

PO Box 1
10 Toft Green
York YO1 7NJ
Helpline: 0845 769 7555

Email: help@alcoholics-anonymous.org.uk
Website: www.alcoholic-anonymous.ork.uk

Alcoholics Anonymous offers a spiritually oriented community of alcoholics who aim to stay sober and, through shared experience and understanding, help other alcoholics to do the same, 'one day at a time' by avoiding that first drink. The essence of the programme involves a 'spiritual awakening' that is achieved by 'working the steps', usually with the guidance of a more experienced member or 'sponsor'.

Al-Anon

61 Great Dover Street
London SE1 4YF
Helpline: 020 7403 0888
Website: www.al-anonuk.org.uk

Al-Anon offers understanding and support for families and friends of problem drinkers. Through group meetings, members receive comfort and understanding and exchange experience, strength, and hope. They learn that there are things that they can do to help themselves and, indirectly, to help the problem drinker. Alateen is for teenagers aged 12 to 17 who are affected by a problem drinker.

Cocaine Anonymous UK

PO Box 46920
London E2 9WF
Helpline: 0800 612 0225 (FOC, 10am–10pm, 7/7)
Website: www.cauk.org.uk

Cocaine Anonymous offers a fellowship of men and women who share their experiences, strength, and hope with one another to recover from their addiction. The only requirement for membership is a desire to stop using cocaine and all other mind-altering substances.

QUIT

20–22 Curtain Road
London EC2A 3NF
Quitline: 0800 00 22 00
Website: www.quit.org.uk

Quit's mission statement is to provide practical help, advice, and support to all smokers who want to stop.

By the same author

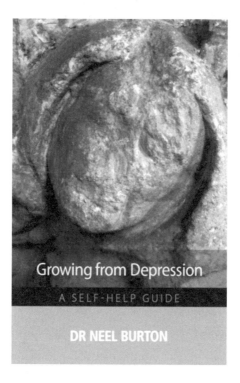

Growing from Depression: A Self-Help Guide

ISBN 978-0-09560353-4-9

...this book is a comprehensive, sympathetic, and thought-provoking guide for those who want to explore their depression in more depth and who are motivated to make long-term changes in their ways of thinking and their lifestyle. It can also be recommended to carers of people with depression and to junior doctors in psychiatry.

The British Journal of Psychiatry

Practical, concise, [this book] does not overwhelm the reader and can be re-read and used as a 'what can I do now?' guide for those affected themselves or carers. The book brings understanding and encourages independent solutions. It is remarkable in its shortness and practicality. Pragmatic yet empathetic.

The British Medical Association

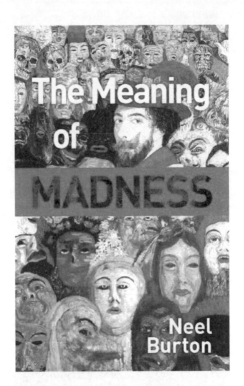

The Meaning of Madness

ISBN 978-0-9560353-0-1

This book proposes to open up the debate on mental disorders, to get people interested and talking, and to get them thinking. For example, what is schizophrenia? Why is it so common? Why does it affect human beings and not animals? What might this tell us about our mind and body, language and creativity, music and religion? What are the boundaries between mental disorder and 'normality'? Is there a relationship between mental disorder and genius? These are some of the difficult but important questions that this book confronts, with the overarching aim of exploring what mental disorders can teach us about human nature and the human condition.

This book is a delight... there is no circumlocution or obliqueness, and the surgical efficiency with which the subjects are addressed makes for maximum comprehension... a really accessible and thorough approach to a complex and often impenetrable subject.

British Neuroscience Association

A life-changing eye-opener.

Reviewer on amazon.co.uk

Index